D0752613

HEALTHY EXCHANG
by JoAnna M. Lund

The Heart Smart Healthy Exchanges® Cookbook

"A valuable resource for patients with heart disease as well as those wishing to take a step toward a heart-healthy lifestyle."

—Debra Hilliard Jones, R.D., L.D.,
Baylor University Medical Center

"I recommend this cookbook to all my cardiac patients, diabetics, athletes, and to those folks who just want to improve overall health. Eat well and enjoy!"

—Maureen M. Kremer, M.S., R.D., L.M.N.T.

The Strong Bones Healthy Exchanges® Cookbook

"An excellent way to incorporate more calcium into your diet while maintaining a low-fat approach to eating."

—Kerry Humes, M.D.,
Women's Health Center, Moline, IL

"I highly recommend [it] to my patients as a nutritious and delicious way to increase their calcium intake."

—Becky Goodell, R.D., L.D.,
Albert Lea Medical Center, Albert Lea, Minnesota

The Diabetic's Healthy Exchanges® Cookbook

"I'm recommending [these recipes] to all my diabetic patients."

—Donna S. Conway, R.N., B.S.N., M.A., C.D.E.

". . . Creative, fun, easy, very tasty . . . my diabetic patients' favorites!"

—Yvonne Guthrie, R.D., C.D.E.

ALSO BY JOANNA M. LUND

The Healthy Exchanges Cookbook
HELP: The Healthy Exchanges Lifetime Plan
Cooking Healthy with a Man in Mind
Cooking Healthy with the Kids in Mind
Diabetic Desserts
Make a Joyful Table
Cooking Healthy Across America
A Potful of Recipes
Another Potful of Recipes
Sensational Smoothies
Hot Off the Grill: The Healthy Exchanges Electric Grilling Cookbook
Cooking Healthy with Splenda
Cooking Healthy with a Microwave
The Diabetic's Healthy Exchanges Cookbook
The Strong Bones Healthy Exchanges Cookbook
The Arthritis Healthy Exchanges Cookbook
The Heart Smart Healthy Exchanges Cookbook
The Cancer Recovery Healthy Exchanges Cookbook
String of Pearls
Family and Friends Cookbook
JoAnna's Kitchen Miracles
When Life Hands You Lemons, Make Lemon Meringue Pie
Cooking Healthy with Soy
Baking Healthy with Splenda
Cooking for Two
Cooking Healthy with a Food Processor
Pizza Anytime
30 Minutes to Mealtime

The
Open Road
Cookbook

A HEALTHY EXCHANGES® COOKBOOK

Healthy Home Cooking . . .
Away from Home

JoAnna M. Lund
with Barbara Alpert

A Perigee Book

A PERIGEE BOOK
Published by the Penguin Group
Penguin Group (USA) Inc.
375 Hudson Street, New York, New York 10014, USA
Penguin Group (Canada), 90 Eglinton Avenue East, Suite 700, Toronto, Ontario M4P 2Y3, Canada
(a division of Pearson Penguin Canada Inc.)
Penguin Books Ltd., 80 Strand, London WC2R 0RL, England
Penguin Group Ireland, 25 St. Stephen's Green, Dublin 2, Ireland (a division of Penguin Books Ltd.)
Penguin Group (Australia), 250 Camberwell Road, Camberwell, Victoria 3124, Australia
(a division of Pearson Australia Group Pty. Ltd.)
Penguin Books India Pvt. Ltd., 11 Community Centre, Panchsheel Park, New Delhi—110 017, India
Penguin Group (NZ), 67 Apollo Drive, Rosedale, North Shore 0745, Auckland, New Zealand
(a division of Pearson New Zealand Ltd.)
Penguin Books (South Africa) (Pty.) Ltd., 24 Sturdee Avenue, Rosebank, Johannesburg 2196,
South Africa

Penguin Books Ltd., Registered Offices: 80 Strand, London WC2R 0RL, England

While the author has made every effort to provide accurate telephone numbers and Internet addresses at
the time of publication, neither the publisher nor the author assumes any responsibility for errors, or for
changes that occur after publication. Further, the publisher does not have any control over and does not
assume any responsibility for author or third-party websites or their content.

For more information about Healthy Exchanges products, contact:
Healthy Exchanges, Inc.
P.O. Box 80
DeWitt, Iowa 52742-0080
(563) 659-8234
www.HealthyExchanges.com

First edition: April 2003

Library of Congress Cataloging-in-Publication Data

Lund, JoAnna M.
    The open road cookbook : a healthy exchanges cookbook : fast and easy recipes for RVers, boaters,
campers, tailgaters—when you want healthy home cooking away from home / JoAnna M. Lund, with
Barbara Alpert.—1st ed.
        p. cm.
    Includes index.
    ISBN 978-0-399-52862-0 (pbk.)
    1. Outdoor cookery. 2. Quick and easy cookery. I. Alpert, Barbara. II. Title.

TX823 .L86 2003
641.5'78—dc21

                                                                                2002035510

PRINTED IN THE UNITED STATES OF AMERICA

10 9 8

PUBLISHER'S NOTE: The recipes contained in this book are to be followed exactly as written. The
publisher is not responsible for your specific health or allergy needs that may require medical
supervision. The publisher is not responsible for any adverse reactions to the recipes contained in this
book.

Most Perigee Books are available at special quantity discounts for bulk purchases for sales promotions,
premiums, fund-raising, or educational use. Special books, or book excerpts, can also be created to fit
specific needs. For details, write: Special Markets, Penguin Group (USA) Inc., 375 Hudson Street, New
York, New York 10014.

This cookbook is dedicated in loving memory to my parents, Jerome and Agnes McAndrews. All the years I was growing up, we lived in a huge old house in Lost Nation, Iowa, where the kitchen was big, but the equipment and storage space were sparse, at best. So I learned firsthand from Mom how to do much with little by stirring in a helping of creativity—be it ingredients or equipment. Daddy was always the analytical thinker and taught my sisters and me to think "outside the box" long before it was popular to do so. I like to think that I'm putting both Mom's and Daddy's talents to good use in these ultra-easy "make do" recipes.

As usual, my mother had the perfect poem for this collection of recipes among the many, many poems she wrote over the years. It really doesn't matter if you're cooking in a motor home, on a boat, while tailgating or picnicking—or even trying to get by in a tiny, cramped apartment galley kitchen—I think you'll enjoy both my recipes and Mom's words.

The Supreme Architect

It isn't so much the house that counts
as the people who live inside.
For houses can burn and tumble down
or be swept away with the tide.
The furniture, too, can go out of style
and become shabby-looking over time.
But, abode shouldn't matter to those in the house;
rather, it's keeping the soul sublime.
For, after this life, when we crumble to dust
as time continues to go endlessly by,
The Supreme Architect, who created this world,
has a mansion waiting for us in the sky.

—Agnes Carrington McAndrews

Contents

Acknowledgments

Just as it's important to choose just the right ingredients when creating "pared-down" recipes, it's vitally important to be surrounded by supportive people when working on deadline for manuscripts. For helping me do my very best when it comes to creating yet another cookbook, I want to thank:

Cliff Lund—my husband. It's been more than ten years since Healthy Exchanges forever changed his life, and I'm amazed that he still delights in taste-testing my new creations every bit as much today as he did when he first took on those duties.

Barbara Alpert—my writing partner. This is our twenty-fourth project together in seven years, and she's still as much a helping hand and listening ear to me as when we first began our collaboration back in 1994. She helps me "season" my words better than if I were the only "cook"!

Shirley Morrow and Rita Ahlers—my typist and my tester. Back in 1991, when Shirley typed my very first recipe, she realized right away that while I'm exceedingly creative, I sure can't spell! Rita has been helping me test recipes since 1995, and she's learned that it doesn't bother me when things go astray under my bed—but when it comes to recipe testing, I'm a perfectionist! All these years and all those recipes—Shirley's probably typed over ten thousand recipes for me, and Rita's tested at least five thousand of them—and they still smile when they come to work here at Timber Ridge Farm!

Coleen O'Shea—my agent. When I told Coleen last year that I was ready to write another book, she made sure everything happened so that I could. She's been doing that for me ever since 1993, when we first met over a piece of my pie!

John Duff—my editor. I am so blessed to have John working on my projects. He never tries to change my Midwest ways, my "common folk" healthy recipes or my "Grandma Moses" style of writing—he just challenges me to meet new goals with each new book. I knew I'd like working with him when he flashed his captivating smile at our first meeting, back in 1994.

God—my creator and my savior. Back in 1991, when I changed

my prayer from what I wanted (a Hollywood skinny body) to what I needed (a real-world healthy body), He blessed me with talents I never dreamed I possessed. Through God all things are possible—from creating recipes to writing books to meeting deadlines!

On the Road—
And on the Path
to Better Health

I'm sure you've noticed the trend, just as I have. We're a nation on the move, eager to experience all that our beautiful country has to offer. Given a choice between staying home and going on the road, we joyfully gas up the van, stock the RV, stuff the tent into its duffel bag, shine the brass on the boat, and spread out the maps on the nearest table or car trunk. When the sun comes up (or often hours before), we're rarin' to go, seat belts buckled, gaze fixed on the highway ahead, exhilarated by the possibilities of seeing someplace new and meeting strangers who'll soon become friends.

I know this as well as anyone, because my husband, Cliff, and I have spent untold hours, days, even weeks on the road during the past ten years. We've toured to promote my cookbooks, driven thousands of miles to visit with our kids and welcome our grandkids, and been thrilled to come face-to-face with the inspiring natural beauty of this land of ours. Even before we began traveling together, Cliff racked up a million miles or more in his years working as a long-distance trucker. So I can speak with authority about this. We Lunds know a lot about living life at sixty-five miles an hour!

Along the way, we've had the genuine pleasure of meeting and sharing meals with wonderful people from every state in the union and even a few foreign countries. We've talked for hours about the way we eat and live on the road for business and pleasure. As they say, no experience is ever wasted, which is a big part of why I decided to write this particular cookbook.

Just because you're living on the road, you don't want to become a prisoner of fast-food restaurants, or a victim of all-day snacking, which is sure to send you back home with a few souvenirs you definitely didn't want: an expanded waistline, fat-clogged arteries, even spotty skin and dull-looking hair. But these are some of the unexpected and distressing side effects that can come with spending time eating and living "on the go."

That said, it doesn't have to be this way. It's not only possible to maintain a healthy lifestyle while traveling, it's much easier than you might think. With some quick and tasty recipes in your tote bag, a well-stocked pantry and RV kitchen (or boat galley), and a commitment to eat and live well away from home, you're ready to make a good thing even better.

Cooking

As Cliff and I began riding into the sunset more and more often in our thirty-two-foot "home away from home," I knew I wanted even quicker and easier recipes for my RV cooking. After all, even though I have most of life's conveniences aboard (including a four-burner stove, oven, microwave, refrigerator, and freezer), do I really want to spend very much of my time cooking? My answer is a resounding NO!

While visiting with other RV-ers, I discovered that they, too, want to cook a little differently when they are traveling up and down the highways of life. At home, with handy garbage disposals and many more cupboards for appliances and supplies, they don't mind the few "extra steps" a recipe requires, even when it means more dishes to wash. (They've got the latest in dishwashers, too!)

But when they are RV-ing, they don't want to bother. Oh, they still want their daily bread to be tasty and healthy, but they also want it to be quick and prepared without much fuss. They need delectable dishes to take to those fun and frequent potlucks at the RV parks, and they want everyone to think that they spent hours preparing them. They want easy recipes for breakfast, lunch, and supper, so they have more time for visiting, reading, playing golf, shopping, sight-seeing, or even taking a well-deserved nap! They want to be able to stock their cupboards once a week and not have to bother stopping at a grocery store again until the following week. They want recipes that call for no more than SIX ingredients, tops—or fewer, if possible. (After all, the more ingredients needed, the more storage space or grocery store stops necessary to fix that dish!) And they want recipes that use canned goods as much as possible because cans store so well. Oh, and they want every dish to taste as delicious as possible.

Sound like an impossible task? Not if you decide to cook in *The Healthy Exchanges Way!* This book is going to teach you how.

Eating

Does this sound familiar? Donuts for breakfast, burgers and fries for lunch, ice cream pops whenever you stop for gas, sugary sodas served all day to thirsty kids, and heavy meals gobbled down too late in the day for good digestion—it's a recipe for disaster, don't you think?

But eating on the go is really about choices, and you've always got the choice to eat healthy, making the best of a situation that appears challenging but doesn't have to be hopeless. You'll feel and look better, and you'll enjoy your journey more, if you plan what you're going to eat—and you build in time to eat it at a table, with place settings, and more than a minute or two to relax.

When we've got plans for an early start, Cliff and I will drink juice and eat cereal before taking to the road. If we're based at a campground or RV park, we'll often enjoy a hot breakfast before heading out. Years of experience—and what we've both learned about good nutrition—tell us that we're bound to have a better day if we fuel ourselves as well as the motor home before putting another mile on the odometer! The great thing about breakfast is it gets your metabolism rolling early, energizes you for the exciting day ahead, and sharpens your reflexes, which makes all the difference for the designated driver.

Like many other traveling couples, we'll regularly dine "al fresco" for lunch, picnicking by the roadside when we spot a nice place to pull over, or setting out our lawn chairs and taking a few minutes to enjoy the scenery before driving the next leg of our journey. Sometimes, lunch is just sandwiches and Diet Mountain Dew, but more often I'll heat up something tasty from the fridge or spoon out a platter of fresh salads on a steamy summer afternoon. It's more refreshing and less harried to stop when you want to, *where* you want to, than worry about finding a convenient restaurant off the highway when hunger pangs hit.

The same is true for dinner, which is why I've provided so many delicious entrees for you to choose from in this book. "Home cooking away from home" is what I call it, and it's good for the soul as well as the body! Taking the time to eat together, either at your table or in some nearby pretty locale, adds so much to the quality of your jaunt across the state or across the country.

Finally, you want to be prepared for those snack attacks that inevitably occur when you're covering lots of miles without a break. Instead of succumbing to candy bars and bags of nuts at a convenience store, you'll be ready for anything with homemade goodies that are truly good—and good for you.

Moving

We've all experienced "creaky body," that uncomfortable sensation of being wedged into the seat of your car for hours on end, then climbing out of the car and feeling cramped and tight-limbed. The more days in a row you'll be spending on the road, the more urgent it is to get moving whenever and wherever you can!

I used to get laughs at my speaking engagements when I shared with my audience that I would "walk the car" when Cliff stopped for gas, but I was telling the truth. I knew I needed the exercise, I always felt better afterward, and if I didn't have access to a gym, a YWCA, or a track, I walked where I could, and when I could—which for me was around and around the car! Did I get any funny looks when people noticed a tall, blond woman doing laps around our dusty vehicle? You bet I did, but I decided not to let it bother me. I knew I was doing something positive for my health, and that gave me courage and confidence to keep on going.

Maybe movie stars and professional athletes can travel with their own trainers and a mobile gym, but that kind of life isn't for the rest of us, and I'm not sure we'd choose it even if we could. But recognizing that we have a choice to take care of ourselves while traveling, and that we have to make our own chance to do so, means being inventive. Finding what works for you may take a few tries, but I'd like to share what some friends have discovered, as well as a few tricks I've tried and liked.

There's been lots written about the need for women in particular to get plenty of weight-bearing exercise as they grow older, primarily to prevent osteoporosis. But walking and striding and other kinds of ambulating also deliver a wonderful aerobic wallop if you do them with enough intensity to break a sweat and get your heart rate up. Whether you choose to walk laps around the deck of your boat or your parked motor home is up to you. But planning exercise breaks is just smart traveling—and making time for special events, like joining a ranger-led hike in a national park, is also a terrific way to stay healthy and see more of the land you're passing through.

Another good idea is lifting weights. I'm not talking about giant dumbbells weighing hundreds of pounds or suggesting you need to pack a steel bench and a barbell in your already crowded RV storage space. But finding a spot for a couple of Dynabands or some five-pound dumbbells is downright doable. If that's more than you can manage on a particular trip, you can still get those muscles moving by using some cans of vegetables or juice as handy temporary weights. I do recommend making this a separate activity from your walking, as recent research suggests that carrying hand weights while aerobic walking can stress the muscles of the wrists and forearms.

What else can you do to get some healthy exercise while traveling? Carry a little gym bag packed with a bathing suit and whatever else you need to enjoy a quick swim. If you're a Y member in your hometown, check to see about reciprocal privileges that permit you to visit other YWCAs around the country. Many national health clubs allow brief visits from out-of-town members, while other clubs invite guests for a few dollars a visit.

I won't deny there are frequently obstacles to getting moving when you're on the road, but attitude is everything—if you are determined to find a way, you'll be surprised what options you'll discover. Not only that, but you're likely to meet some great people while pounding the pavement or stroking down a lane in a new pool!

Resting

So often, we live our lives at a breakneck pace, vowing to drive straight through from New York to Orlando to get the most time at Disney World we can, or else we plan journeys that cover a dozen states in a week, allowing for travel time, eating breaks, high points sight-seeing—but not a reasonable amount of rest. It seems that we define vacation by how much we can cram into a few days off from work or school, but in our haste to see and taste and encounter a whole new world, we forget that getting enough rest is a requirement for good health, not a luxury.

Most of the people who've heard me speak know that I'm an early riser, that I'm usually out of bed a couple of hours before sunrise. I like that early-morning time for walking, for thinking, for writing, and for praying before I start my new day. When Cliff and I travel, he likes to hit the road before traffic gets heavy—again, a habit developed during his years as a long-distance truck driver. But in order to do this and not burn out, we head off to sleep at a reasonable hour. So we don't often watch the ten o'clock news or stay up for one more late movie. In order to get the most out of our days, we make the most of our nights, too.

If travel noise is a problem for you, invest in one of those "hummers" that lulls you to sleep to the sound of ocean waves; if it's often too light outside, experiment with darker window shades or even an eye mask. And if you have trouble sleeping in an unfamiliar bed, bring a pillow or light quilt from home that turns every bedroom into a cozy, comforting, restful oasis.

Your body requires a certain amount of rest, whether you're lying in a sleeping bag in a tent in Yosemite or rocked gently to sleep while lake breezes filter through the screen of your porthole. Giving yourself the gift of true relaxation and a chance to dream about all the tomorrows to come is not only a good healthy choice but a simple way to make a good trip one to remember and cherish forever.

Planning

For some of us, travel is the ultimate enjoyable activity, but if you're touring with your kids, traveling on business, or covering a lot of unfamiliar territory, you know the kind of stress and strain such a trip can produce. There's a four-letter-word that can spell the difference between chaos and comfort, between misery and a marvelous time. To have the best possible experience each time you hit the road, you need to PLAN.

Well, yes, you may say, we've got plenty of maps—but has anyone organized them so it takes a second to find the one you need when it's ten P.M. and you may have missed your exit? Have you stocked the glove compartment with a flashlight and extra batteries so you can read the map in case your car light is on the blink? Have you checked handy Websites in and around your destinations and printed out a list of family-friendly restaurants, or phone numbers of late-night pharmacies (if you often require medical supplies) and pet hospitals (if you're accompanied by your beloved but aging dog)?

Even if your personal travel style has been free-spirited, even haphazard, up to now, you'll soon discover that some extra planning ahead can be the key to the smoothest possible vacation. You'll see that I've provided a list of how to stock your travel kitchen and pantry before you leave home. I know you can shop on the road, but why leave it to the last minute, when the sun is out, the kids are hungry, and you'd rather be playing golf?

Brainstorm with your travel companions—kids and adults alike—about what you may want or need to carry with you. If you're a fan of certain products that may not be available where you're heading, pack the car! (I remember a couple who departed for a cross-country journey with a dozen bags of bagel chips and gallons of spring water. They'd recently read a *People* magazine article about a stranded couple who survived days in the woods because they'd had the foresight to pack plenty of food in their backseat!)

Planning is even more important when you're committed to living a healthy lifestyle, especially when you're miles from home. I heard a motivational speaker once say, "If you fail to plan, you plan to fail." Those are strong sentiments, but the philosophy behind them makes good common sense. By organizing yourself before you put "pedal to the metal," you increase the odds of having the best time ever!

Breathing

This is sort of a funny category, but when I was listing topics to share with you, this word came to mind. I'm not talking about the inhale/exhale kind of breathing, but instead the idea of "breathing room." To me, this means not scheduling yourself within an inch of your life, so that the priority becomes how many miles a day you can rack up or how many sights and states you can check off a list. Giving yourself and your loved ones breathing room means taking the time to really enjoy each hour, each day, each new place, and each new person.

I know it's not always easy, especially when you're on the road for business rather than pleasure. But the price of not doing it, not taking care of yourself in this way, is too often burnout. In a worst-case scenario, you may even endanger yourself and others by driving too many hours in a row without sufficient food or rest.

I've come to treasure time in recent months as never before. Facing a health crisis brings an amazing clarity to every situation, and while I'm not suggesting any of us want to invite illness into our lives, I've learned some valuable lessons while coping with my recent diagnosis of breast cancer. Now, when we travel, we have to leave a little more time, cover a little less distance, make allowances for different needs than we once did. But a positive side effect of making those changes is that we find we enjoy our journeys more, cherish the time spent together both in and out of the car, and make a point of relishing each meal, each beautiful sight, and each friendly encounter with someone we've just met.

Breathing also means finding the joy in quiet times together, when no words are necessary. You're surrounded by the ones you love, and you simply sigh with pleasure. Isn't life wonderful?

Detours

No, I'm not talking about the kind that are caused by miles of road construction (or de-struction, as we sometimes call it!). I mean the kind of detour you *choose* to take, the side trips and pleasant excursions that are often not part of the big picture but turn out to be what is most remembered at journey's end. After years of traveling all over the country, I've learned a lesson worth passing along—go on the wild-goose chase in search of the legendary diner whose pies make a trucker grin with delight, take the dirt road to look for the dusty ghost town that was once home to a gold rush, and "waste" a morning or afternoon at a dozen garage sales along a stretch of road that many drive but too few stop on for a visit and a glass of lemonade. It's these detours, these surprises, that create the most unforgettable memories. Maybe you'll pause for dinner at a vintage hotel where your husband once dined during basic training; perhaps you'll discover a small-town pet show where the grand prize is offered for the "dog with the waggiest tail!" Be open to these side trips as often as you can, and you'll be happy you did!

Reaching Out

In the end, it's the people we remember most.

They're the true reward for traveling, the strangers who become friends, the families who have kids just the same ages as ours. They share our suppers at picnic tables in campgrounds, provide jumper cables when an RV battery dies, join in an impromptu sing-along when someone pulls out a guitar, and deepen our appreciation of the precious world we've been given.

I feel sometimes as if I've met a million wonderful people "on the go." I know that with my QVC appearances and PBS series, I've reached out to even more than that, and I'm grateful for the opportunity. But whether I'm visiting with a few or a multitude, I appreciate the chance to be a part of their lives and to welcome them into mine, even if just for a few minutes or hours. No matter how tired we are or how many miles we've traveled, we've tried to make time for these important connections—for they make life especially worth living! And by creating meals that people everywhere can share, I feel I'm contributing to all those glorious occasions when friends dine and chat and have a truly great time together!

Hitting the Road

While I believe this collection of survival information and "common folk" healthy recipes will be appreciated by everyone who camps (from tents to fold ups to cabins), it's especially intended for those vast, untold numbers of fifty-plus, "young-at-heart" RV-ers who want to enjoy life as they make their personal journeys toward good health. As you travel around at your own pace, you want and need to eat well and enjoy each repast. These recipes are as quick and tasty as they are healthy, and that makes lifelong good sense. Just because we take vacations from our everyday routines doesn't mean that we should take vacations from our healthy eating habits too!

To make life on the road even easier, I've included advice on how to stock up your kitchen and pantry. I'm also sharing my JoAnna's "Driver's Dozen" Traveling Cook's Tips to help you along the way. After cooking up a storm with the recipes in this collection, you may be wondering why you didn't take to the road sooner. The only thing I could do to help you more would be to stop by and do your dishes!

Even if you only get two weeks' vacation a year and cook dinner most nights in a cramped apartment kitchen, *The Open Road Cookbook* is geared for you, too. And if you're lucky enough to prepare meals in a big country kitchen, imagine how easy these recipes will be for you as well.

Cliff and I wish you **Happy Healthy Trails**—and hope to see you on the road!

Food Exchanges and Weight Loss Choices™

If you've ever been on one of the national weight-loss programs like Weight Watchers or Diet Center, you've already been introduced to the concept of measured portions of different food groups that make up your daily food plan. If you are not familiar with such a system of weight-loss choices or exchanges, here's a brief explanation. (If you want or need more detailed information, you can write to the American Dietetic Association or the American Diabetes Association for comprehensive explanations.)

The idea of food exchanges is to divide foods into basic food groups. The foods in each group are measured in servings that have comparable values. These groups include Proteins/Meats, Breads/Starches, Vegetables, Fats, Fruits, Fat-Free Milk, Free Foods, and Optional Calories.

Each choice or exchange included in a particular group has about the same number of calories and a similar carbohydrate, protein, and fat content as the other foods in that group. Because any food on a particular list can be "exchanged" for any other food in that group, it makes sense to call the food groups *exchanges* or *choices*.

I like to think we are also "exchanging" bad habits and food choices for good ones!

By using Weight Loss Choices or exchanges you can choose from a variety of foods without having to calculate the nutrient value of each one. This makes it easier to include a wide variety of foods in your daily menus and gives you the opportunity to tailor your choices to your unique appetite.

If you want to lose weight, you should consult your physician or other weight-control expert regarding the number of servings that would be best for you from each food group. Since men generally require more calories than women, and since the requirements for growing children and teenagers differ from those of adults, the right number of exchanges for any one person is a personal decision.

I have included a suggested plan of weight-loss choices in the pages following the exchange lists. It's a program I used to lose 130 pounds, and it's the one I still follow today.

(If you are a diabetic or have been diagnosed with heart problems, it is best to meet with your physician before using this or any other food program or recipe collection.)

Food Group Weight Loss Choices™/Exchanges

Not all food group exchanges are alike. The ones that follow are for anyone who's interested in weight loss or maintenance. If you are a diabetic, you should check with your health-care provider or dietitian to get the information you need to help you plan your diet. Diabetic exchanges are calculated by the American Diabetic Association, and information about them is provided in *The Diabetic's Healthy Exchanges Cookbook* (Perigee Books).

Every Healthy Exchanges recipe provides calculations in three ways:

- Weight Loss Choices/Exchanges
- Calories, Fat, Protein, Carbohydrates, and Fiber in grams, and Sodium and Calcium in milligrams
- Diabetic Exchanges calculated for me by a registered dietitian

Healthy Exchanges recipes can help you eat well and recover your health, whatever your health concerns may be. Please take a few minutes to review the exchange lists and the suggestions that follow on how to count them. You have lots of great eating in store for you!

Proteins
Meat, poultry, seafood, eggs, cheese, and legumes.
One exchange of Protein is approximately 60 calories. Examples of one Protein choice or exchange:

1 ounce cooked weight of lean meat, poultry, or seafood
2 ounces white fish
1½ ounces 97% fat-free ham
1 egg (limit to no more than 4 per week)
¼ cup egg substitute
3 egg whites
¾ ounce reduced-fat cheese
½ cup fat-free cottage cheese
2 ounces cooked or ¾ ounces uncooked dry beans
1 tablespoon peanut butter (also count 1 fat exchange)

Breads

Breads, crackers, cereals, grains, and starchy vegetables. One exchange of Bread is approximately 80 calories. Examples of one Bread choice or exchange:

1 slice bread or 2 slices reduced-calorie bread (40 calories or less)
1 roll, any type (1 ounce)
½ cup cooked pasta or ¾ ounce uncooked (scant ½ cup)
½ cup cooked rice or 1 ounce uncooked (⅓ cup)
3 tablespoons flour
¾ ounce cold cereal
½ cup cooked hot cereal or ¾ ounce uncooked (2 tablespoons)
½ cup corn (kernels or cream-style) or peas
4 ounces white potato, cooked, or 5 ounces uncooked
3 ounces sweet potato, cooked, or 4 ounces uncooked
3 cups air-popped popcorn
7 fat-free crackers (¾ ounce)
3 (2½-inch squares) graham crackers
2 (¾-ounce) rice cakes or 6 mini
1 tortilla, any type (6-inch diameter)

Fruits

All fruits and fruit juices. One exchange of Fruit is approximately 60 calories. Examples of one Fruit choice or exchange:

1 small apple or ½ cup slices
1 small orange
½ medium banana
¾ cup berries (except strawberries and cranberries)
1 cup strawberries or cranberries

½ cup canned fruit, packed in fruit juice or rinsed well
2 tablespoons raisins
1 tablespoon spreadable fruit spread
½ cup apple juice (4 fluid ounces)
½ cup orange juice (4 fluid ounces)
½ cup applesauce

Fat-Free Milk

Milk, buttermilk, and yogurt. One exchange of Fat-Free Milk is approximately 90 calories. Examples of one Fat-Free Milk choice or exchange:

1 cup fat-free milk
½ cup evaporated fat-free milk
1 cup low-fat buttermilk
¾ cup plain fat-free yogurt
⅓ cup nonfat dry milk powder

Vegetables

All fresh, canned, or frozen vegetables other than the starchy vegetables. One exchange of Vegetable is approximately 30 calories. Examples of one Vegetable choice or exchange:

½ cup vegetable
¼ cup tomato sauce
1 medium fresh tomato
½ cup vegetable juice
1 cup shredded lettuce or cabbage

Fats

Margarine, mayonnaise, vegetable oils, salad dressings, olives, and nuts. One exchange of Fat is approximately 40 calories. Examples of one Fat choice or exchange:

1 teaspoon margarine or 2 teaspoons reduced-calorie margarine
1 teaspoon butter
1 teaspoon vegetable oil
1 teaspoon mayonnaise or 2 teaspoons reduced-calorie mayonnaise
1 teaspoon peanut butter
1 ounce olives
¼ ounce pecans or walnuts

Free Foods

Foods that do not provide nutritional value but are used to enhance the taste of foods are included in the Free Foods group. Examples of these are spices, herbs, extracts, vinegar, lemon juice, mustard, Worcestershire sauce, and soy sauce. Cooking sprays and artificial sweeteners used in moderation are also included in this group. However, you'll see that I include the caloric value of artificial sweeteners in the Optional Calories of the recipes.

You may occasionally see a recipe that lists "free food" as part of the portion. According to the published exchange lists, a free food contains fewer than 20 calories per serving. Two or three servings per day of free foods/drinks are usually allowed in a meal plan.

Optional Calories

Foods that do not fit into any other group but are used in moderation in recipes are included in Optional Calories. Foods that are counted in this way include sugar-free gelatin and puddings, fat-free mayonnaise and dressings, reduced-calorie whipped toppings, reduced-calorie syrups and jams, chocolate chips, coconut, and canned broth.

Sliders™

These are 80 Optional Calorie increments that do not fit into any particular category. You can choose which food group to *slide* these into. It is wise to limit this selection to approximately three to four per day to ensure the best possible nutrition for your body while still enjoying an occasional treat.

Sliders may be used in either of the following ways:

1. If you have consumed all your Protein, Bread, Fruit, or Fat-Free Milk Weight Loss Choices for the day, and you want to eat additional foods from those food groups, you simply use a Slider. It's what I call "healthy horse trading." Remember that Sliders may not be traded for choices in the Vegetables or Fats food groups.

2. Sliders may also be deducted from your Optional Calories for the day or week. One-quarter Slider equals 20 Optional Calories; ½ Slider equals 40 Optional Calories; ¾ Slider equals 60 Optional Calories; and 1 Slider equals 80 Optional Calories.

Healthy Exchanges®
Weight Loss Choices™

My original Healthy Exchanges program of Weight Loss Choices was based on an average daily total of 1,400 to 1,600 calories per day. That was what I determined was right for my needs, and for those of most women. Because men require additional calories (about 1,600 to 1,900), here are my suggested plans for women and men. *(If you require more or fewer calories, please revise this plan to meet your individual needs.)*

Each day, women should plan to eat:

2 Fat-Free Milk choices, 90 calories each
2 Fat choices, 40 calories each
3 Fruit choices, 60 calories each
4 Vegetable choices or more, 30 calories each
5 Protein choices, 60 calories each
5 Bread choices, 80 calories each

Each day, men should plan to eat:

2 Fat-Free Milk choices, 90 calories each
4 Fat choices, 40 calories each
3 Fruit choices, 60 calories each
4 Vegetable choices or more, 30 calories each
6 Protein choices, 60 calories each
7 Bread choices, 80 calories each

Young people should follow the program for men but add 1 Fat-Free Milk choice for a total of 3 servings.

You may also choose to add up to 100 Optional Calories per day, and up to 21 to 28 Sliders per week at 80 calories each. If you choose to include more Sliders in your daily or weekly totals, deduct those 80 calories from your Optional Calorie "bank."

A word about Sliders: These are to be counted toward your totals after you have used your allotment of choices of Fat-Free Milk, Protein, Bread, and Fruit for the day. By "sliding" an additional choice into one of these groups, you can meet your individual needs for that day. Sliders are especially helpful when traveling, stressed-out, eating out, or for special events. I often use mine so I can enjoy my favorite Healthy Exchanges desserts. Vegetables are not to be counted as Sliders. Enjoy as many Vegetable choices as you need to feel satisfied. Because we want to limit our fat intake to moderate amounts, additional Fat choices should not be counted as Sliders. If you choose to include more fat on an *occasional* basis, count the extra choices as Optional Calories.

Keep a daily food diary of your Weight Loss Choices, checking off what you eat as you go. If, at the end of the day, your required selections are not 100 percent accounted for, but you have done the best you can, go to bed with a clear conscience. There will be days when you have ¼ Fruit or ½ Bread left over. What are you going to do—eat two slices of an orange or half a slice of bread and throw the rest out? I always say, "Nothing in life comes out exact." Just do the best you can . . . *the best you can.*

Try to drink at least eight 8-ounce glasses of water a day. Water truly is the "nectar" of good health.

As a little added insurance, I take a multi-vitamin each day. It's not essential, but if my day's worth of well-planned meals "bites the dust" when unexpected events intrude on my regular routine, my body still gets its vital nutrients.

The calories listed in each group of choices are averages. Some choices within each group may be higher or lower, so it's important to select a variety of different foods instead of eating the same three or four all the time.

Use your Optional Calories! They are what I call "life's little extras." They make all the difference in how you enjoy your food and appreciate the variety available to you. Yes, we can get by without them, but do you really want to? Keep in mind that you should be using all your daily Weight Loss Choices first to ensure you are getting the basics of good nutrition. But I guarantee that Optional Calories will keep you from feeling deprived—and help you reach your weight-loss goals.

JoAnna's Ten Commandments of Successful Cooking

A very important part of any journey is knowing where you are going and the best way to get there. If you plan and prepare before you start to cook, you should reach meal time with foods to write home about!

1. **Read the entire recipe from start to finish** and be sure you understand the process involved. Check that you have all the equipment you will need *before* you begin.

2. **Check the ingredient list** and be sure you have *everything* and in the amounts required. Keep cooking sprays handy—while they're not listed as ingredients, I use them all the time (just a quick squirt!).

3. **Set out *all the ingredients and equipment needed*** to prepare the recipe on the counter near you *before* you start. Remember that old saying *A stitch in time saves nine?* It applies in the kitchen, too.

4. **Do as much advance preparation as possible** before actually cooking. Chop, cut, grate, or do whatever is needed to prepare the ingredients and have them ready before you start to mix. Turn the oven on at least ten minutes before putting food in to bake, to allow the oven to preheat to the proper temperature.

5. **Use a kitchen timer** to tell you when the cooking or baking time is up. Because stove temperatures vary slightly by manufacturer, you may want to set your timer for five min-

utes less than the suggested time just to prevent overcooking. Check the progress of your dish at that time, then decide if you need the additional minutes or not.

6. **Measure carefully.** Use glass measures for liquids and metal or plastic cups for dry ingredients. My recipes are based on standard measurements. Unless I tell you it's a scant or full cup, measure the cup level.

7. **For best results, follow the recipe instructions exactly.** Feel free to substitute ingredients that *don't tamper* with the basic chemistry of the recipe, but be sure to leave key ingredients alone. For example, you could substitute sugar-free instant chocolate pudding for sugar-free instant butterscotch pudding, but if you used a six-serving package when a four-serving package was listed in the ingredients, or you used instant when cook-and-serve is required, you won't get the right result.

8. **Clean up as you go.** It is much easier to wash a few items at a time than to face a whole counter of dirty dishes later. The same is true for spills on the counter or floor.

9. **Be careful about doubling or halving a recipe.** Though many recipes can be altered successfully to serve more or fewer people, *many cannot.* This is especially true when it comes to spices and liquids. If you try to double a recipe that calls for 1 teaspoon pumpkin-pie spice, for example, and you double the spice, you may end up with a too-spicy taste. I usually suggest increasing spices or liquid by 1½ times when doubling a recipe. If it tastes a little bland to you, you can increase the spice to 1¾ times the original amount the next time you prepare the dish. Remember: You can always add more, but you can't take it out after it's stirred in.

   The same is true with liquid ingredients. If you wanted to **triple** a main dish recipe because you were planning to serve a crowd, you might think you should use three times as much of every ingredient. Don't, or you could end up with soup instead! If the original recipe calls for 1¾ cup tomato sauce, I'd suggest using 3½ cups when you **triple** the recipe (or 2¾ cups if you **double** it). You'll still have a good-tasting dish that won't run all over the plate.

10. **Write your reactions next to each recipe once you've served it.**

Yes, that's right, I'm giving you permission to write in this book. It's yours, after all. Ask yourself: Did everyone like it? Did you have to add another half teaspoon of chili seasoning to please your family, who like to live on the spicier side of the street? You may even want to rate the recipe on a scale of 1 ☆ to 4 ☆, depending on what you thought of it. (Four stars would be the top rating—and I hope you'll feel that way about many of my recipes.) Jotting down your comments while they are fresh in your mind will help you personalize the recipe to your own taste the next time you prepare it.

JoAnna's "Driver's Dozen" Traveling Cook's Tips

1. **Precook some food in your "real" kitchen before you leave home.**

   Boil a half dozen potatoes, brown some extra lean ground beef, hard-boil a few eggs, roast some chicken, beef, or pork. Freeze the meats in serving size packages. Put the potatoes in a covered container. Mark the hard-boiled eggs with an X so you can tell them apart from raw ones.

2. **Pre-chop your vegetables.**

   This is a real help when you're ready for a snack and your home is moving 65 miles an hour down a winding highway. It also speeds up preparation time when you're fixing supper.

3. **Pick your times and places to do "prep" cooking when you're on the road.**

   If it's raining, so you can't be out walking or sight-seeing, boil some more eggs or potatoes to get you through the next few days. That way, when the sun does come out, you're free to enjoy it. If it's too hot to be outside and you're sitting in your air-conditioned living room reading or writing "wish you were here" notes, stick a roast in the slow cooker or oven to bake away while you are there to tend to it.

4. **Non-dairy fat-free creamer mixed with nonfat dry milk powder and water tastes like cream on your breakfast cereal.**

It will keep longer than regular milk, especially if you store both the creamer and the dry milk powder in plastic containers in your refrigerator.

5. **Crackers can be used as bread substitutes some of the time.**

   Better still, they won't go stale on you, as long as you store them in an airtight container. Even a week of rainy days won't make them soggy!

6. **Store your flour, instant coffee, and tea in plastic containers.**

   Mark them with masking tape and a bright red marking pen, and you won't have to open every one to find just what you are looking for.

7. **Store your "extra" cans of vegetables, meats, and fruits in boxes under the dinette seats.**

   Just make sure you check your bounty before making your next shopping list—or you're likely to end up with too much of a good thing!

8. **Put ice cubes in a couple of gallon size resealable storage bags and store in your RV freezer.**

   When you want to break them apart, all you have to do is hit the bag against the counter and you have ice ready for your drink. Just refill your bag at the soda fountain dispenser when the "chauffeur" stops for gas. Remember to offer to pay for the ice (usually it won't be more than 50 cents—but that's a lot cheaper and more convenient than the large bags of ice cubes found in most convenience stores).

9. **"Cool Whip Light" containers are the perfect choice for storing leftovers.**

   Don't feel you have to purchase color-coded sets of plastic storage containers to have an organized kitchen. By recycling store-bought ones, you can put the money you save toward mementos from your journey.

10. **If you've got an electrical outlet on the outside of your RV, move the "kitchen" outside in pleasant weather.**

    Plug in your electric skillet or grill when it's time to fix dinner, and you won't have to miss out on enjoying a summer sunset.

11. **Double your counter space by using a cutting board that fits right over your sink.**

    I've seen some that let you rinse your veggies and slice them right on the same well-designed board. Other "tight space" solutions: install additional storage bins that go under cabinets; use disposable serving plates and bowls instead of crowding large, rarely-used items into corners and closets; hang what you can on the wall or from the ceiling—spice rack, kitchen tools, collapsible bins for fruits and veggies. (Just make sure you use sturdy hooks and fasteners that can't be jarred loose by bumps or sudden stops!)

12. **Keep revising what works for you by keeping a kitchen journal.**

    When you packed for your last trip, did you bring along your countertop electric grill and then discover that you used it only once or twice? Did you stock up on canned corn and then eat mostly fresh ears from roadside stands? What you need in a traveling kitchen will likely vary from season to season, year to year, and even depending on who your traveling companions are! By making notes about what works and what doesn't, you can design a layout and pantry shopping list that will make your trip the best possible.

Help Me Cook Healthy: My Best Healthy Exchanges® Cooking Tips

Measurements, General Cooking Tips, and Basic Ingredients

The word *moderation* best describes **my use of fats, sugar substitutes,** and **sodium** in these recipes. Wherever possible, I've used cooking spray for sautéing and for browning meats and vegetables. I also use reduced-calorie margarine and fat-free mayonnaise and salad dressings. Lean ground turkey *or* ground beef can be used in the recipes. Just be sure whatever you choose is at least *90 percent lean.*

Sugar Substitutes

I've also included **small amounts of sugar substitutes as the sweetening agent** in many of the recipes. I don't drink a hundred cans of soda a day or eat enough artificially sweetened foods in a 24-hour time period to be troubled by sugar substitutes. But if this is a concern of yours and you *do not* need to watch your sugar intake, you can always replace the sugar substitutes with processed sugar and the sugar-free products with regular ones.

I created my recipes knowing they would also be used by hypo-glycemics, diabetics, and those concerned about triglycerides. If you choose to use sugar instead, be sure to count the additional calories.

A word of caution when cooking with **sugar substitutes:** Use **sucralose-** or **saccharin**-based sweeteners when **heating or baking.** In recipes that **don't require heat, aspartame** (known as NutraSweet) works well in uncooked dishes but leaves an aftertaste in baked products.

Splenda and **Sugar Twin** are my best choices for sugar substitutes. They measure like sugar, you can cook and bake with them, they're inexpensive, and they are easily poured from their boxes. (If you can't find **Splenda** in your store yet, try their Website: http://www.splenda.com to order directly.)

Many of my recipes for quick breads, muffins, and cakes include a package of sugar-free instant pudding mix, which is sweetened with NutraSweet. Yet we've been told that NutraSweet breaks down under heat. I've tested my recipes again and again, and here's what I've found: baking with a NutraSweet product sold for home sweetening doesn't work, but baking with NutraSweet-sweetened instant pudding mixes turns out great. I choose not to question why this is, but continue to use these products in creating my Healthy Exchanges recipes.

How much sweetener is the right amount? I use pourable Splenda, Sugar Twin, Brown Sugar Twin, and Sprinkle Sweet in my recipes because they measure just like sugar. What could be easier? I also use them because they work wonderfully in cooked and baked products.

If you are using a brand other than these, you need to check the package to figure out how much of your sweetener will equal what's called for in the recipe.

If you choose to use real sugar or brown sugar, then you would use the same amount the recipe lists for pourable Splenda, Sugar Twin, or Brown Sugar Twin.

You'll see that I list only the specific brands when the recipe preparation involves heat. In a salad or other recipe that doesn't require cooking, I will list the ingredient as "sugar substitute to equal

2 tablespoons sugar." You can then use any sweetener you choose—Equal, Sweet'N Low, Sweet Ten, or any other aspartame-based sugar substitute. Just check the label so you'll be using the right amount to equal those 2 tablespoons of sugar. Or, if you choose, you can use regular sugar.

With Healthy Exchanges recipes, the "sweet life" is the only life for me!

Pan Sizes

I'm often asked why I use an **8-by-8-inch baking dish** in my recipes. It's for portion control. If the recipe says it serves 4, just cut down the center, turn the dish, and cut again. Like magic, there's your serving. Also, if this is the only recipe you are preparing requiring an oven, the square dish fits into a tabletop toaster oven easily and energy can be conserved.

While many of my recipes call for an 8-by-8-inch baking dish, others ask for a 9-by-9-inch cake pan. If you don't have a 9-inch-square pan, is it all right to use your 8-inch dish instead? In most cases, the small difference in the size of these two pans won't significantly affect the finished product, so until you can get your hands on the right size pan, go ahead and use your baking dish.

However, since the 8-inch dish is usually made of glass, and the 9-inch cake pan is made of metal, you will want to adjust the baking temperature. If you're using a glass baking dish in a recipe that calls for a 9-inch pan, be sure to lower your baking temperature by 15 degrees *or* check your finished product at least 6 to 8 minutes before the specified baking time is over.

But it really is worthwhile to add a 9-by-9-inch pan to your collection, and if you're going to be baking lots of my Healthy Exchanges cakes, you'll definitely use it frequently. A cake baked in this pan will have a better texture, and the servings will be a little larger. Just think of it—an 8-by-8-inch pan produces 64 square inches of dessert, while a 9-by-9-inch pan delivers 81 square inches. Those 17 extra inches are too tasty to lose!

To make life even easier, **whenever a recipe calls for ounce measurements** (other than raw meats) I've included the closest cup equivalent. I need to use my scale daily when creating recipes, so I've measured for you at the same time.

Freezing Leftovers

Most of the recipes are for **4 to 8 servings.** If you don't have that many to feed, do what I do: freeze individual portions. Then all you have to do is choose something from the freezer and take it to work for lunch or have your evening meals prepared in advance for the week. In this way, I always have something on hand that is both good to eat and good for me.

Unless a recipe includes hard-boiled eggs, cream cheese, mayonnaise, or a raw vegetable or fruit, **the leftovers should freeze well.** (I've marked recipes that freeze well with the symbol of a **snow-flake ❄** .)This includes most of the cream pies. Divide any recipe up into individual servings and freeze for your own "TV" dinners.

Another good idea is **cutting leftover pie into individual pieces and freezing each one separately** in a small resealable freezer bag. Once you've cut the pie into portions, place them on a cookie sheet and put it in the freezer for 15 minutes. That way, the creamy topping won't get smashed and your pie will keep its shape.

When you want to thaw a piece of pie for yourself, you don't have to thaw the whole pie. You can practice portion control at the same time, and it works really well for brown-bag lunches. Just pull a piece out of the freezer on your way to work and by lunchtime you will have a wonderful dessert waiting for you.

Why do I so often recommend freezing leftover desserts? One reason is that if you leave baked goods made with sugar substitute out on the counter for more than a day or two, they get moldy. Sugar is a preservative and retards the molding process. It's actually what's called an *antimicrobial agent*, meaning it works against microbes such as molds, bacteria, fungi, and yeasts that grow in foods and can cause food poisoning. Both sugar and salt work as antimicrobial agents to withdraw water from food. Since microbes can't grow without water, food protected in this way doesn't spoil.

So what do we do if we don't want our muffins to turn moldy, but we also don't want to use sugar because of the excess carbohydrates and calories? Freeze them! Just place each muffin or individually sliced bread serving into a resealable sandwich bag, seal, and toss into your freezer. Then, whenever you want one for a snack or a meal, you can choose to let it thaw naturally or "zap" it in the microwave. If you know that baked goods will be eaten within a day or two, packaging them in a sealed plastic container and storing in the refrigerator will do the trick.

Unless I specify **"covered" for simmering or baking**, prepare my recipes **uncovered**. Occasionally you will read a recipe that asks you to cover a dish for a time, then to uncover, so read the directions carefully to avoid confusion—and to get the best results.

Cooking Spray

Low-fat cooking spray is another blessing in a Healthy Exchanges kitchen. It's currently available in three flavors:

- **OLIVE OIL or GARLIC FLAVORED** when cooking Mexican, Italian, or Greek dishes

- **BUTTER or LEMON FLAVORED** when a hint of butter or lemon is desired

- **REGULAR** for everything else

A quick spray of butter flavored makes air-popped popcorn a low-fat taste treat, or try it as a butter substitute on steaming-hot corn on the cob. One light spray of the skillet when browning meat will convince you that you're using "old-fashioned fat," and a quick coating of the casserole dish before you add the ingredients will make serving easier and cleanup quicker.

Baking Times

Sometimes I give you a range as a **baking time**, such as 22 to 28 minutes. Why? Because every kitchen, every stove, and every chef's cooking technique is slightly different. On a hot and humid day in Iowa, the optimum cooking time won't be the same as on a cold, dry day. Some stoves bake hotter than the temperature setting indicates; other stoves bake cooler. Electric ovens usually are more temperamental than gas ovens. If you place your baking pan on a lower shelf, the temperature is warmer than if you place it on a higher shelf. If you stir the mixture more vigorously than I do, you could affect the required baking time by a minute or more.

The best way to gauge the heat of your particular oven is to purchase an oven temperature gauge that hangs in the oven. These can be found in any discount store or kitchen equipment store, and if you're going to be cooking and baking regularly, it's a good idea to own one. Set the oven to 350 degrees and when the oven indicates that it has reached that temperature, check the reading on the gauge. If it's less than 350 degrees, you know your oven cooks cooler, and you need to add a few minutes to the cooking time *or* set your oven at a higher temperature. If it's more than 350 degrees, then your oven is warmer and you need to subtract a few minutes from the cooking time. In any event, always treat the suggested baking time as approximate. Check on your baked product at the earliest suggested time. You can always continue baking a few minutes more if needed, but you can't unbake it once you've cooked it too long.

Miscellaneous Ingredients and Tips

I use reduced-sodium **canned chicken broth** in place of dry bouillon to lower the sodium content. The intended flavor is still present in the prepared dish. As a reduced-sodium beef broth is not currently available (at least not in DeWitt, Iowa), I use the canned regular beef broth. The sodium content is still lower than regular dry bouillon.

Whenever **cooked rice or pasta** is an ingredient, follow the package directions, but eliminate the salt and/or margarine called for. This helps lower the sodium and fat content. It tastes just fine; trust me on this.

Here's another tip: When **cooking rice or noodles**, why not cook extra "for the pot"? After you use what you need, store leftover rice in a covered container (where it will keep for a couple of days). With noodles like spaghetti or macaroni, first rinse and drain as usual, then measure out what you need. Put the leftovers in a bowl covered with water, then store in the refrigerator, covered, until they're needed. Then, measure out what you need, rinse and drain them, and they're ready to go.

Does your **pita bread** often tear before you can make a sandwich? Here's my tip to make it open easily: cut the bread in half, put the halves in the microwave for about 15 seconds, and they will open up by themselves. *Voilà!*

When **chunky salsa** is listed as an ingredient, I leave the degree of "heat" up to your personal taste. In our house, I'm considered a wimp. I go for the "mild" while Cliff prefers "extra-hot." How do we compromise? I prepare the recipe with mild salsa because he can always add a spoonful or two of the hotter version to his serving, but I can't enjoy the dish if it's too spicy for me.

You can make purchased **fat-free salad dressings** taste **more**

like the "real thing" by adding a small amount of fat-free mayonnaise and a pinch of sugar substitute to the diet dressing. Start with 2 tablespoons of salad dressing (such as Ranch), add 1 teaspoon fat-free mayo and sugar substitute to equal ½ teaspoon sugar. Mix well and spoon over your salad. Unless you remind yourself you're eating the fat-free version, you may just fool yourself into thinking you reached for the high-fat counterpart instead!

Milk, Yogurt, and More

Take it from me—nonfat dry milk powder is great! I *do not* use it for drinking, but I *do* use it for cooking. Three good reasons why:

1. It is very **inexpensive**.

2. It does not **sour** because you use it only as needed. Store the box in your refrigerator or freezer and it will keep almost forever.

3. You can easily **add extra calcium** to just about any recipe without added liquid.

I consider nonfat dry milk powder one of Mother Nature's modern-day miracles of convenience. But do purchase a good national name brand (I like Carnation), and keep it fresh by proper storage.

I've said many times, "Give me my mixing bowl, my wire whisk, and a box of nonfat dry milk powder, and I can conquer the world!" Here are some of my favorite ways to use dry milk powder:

1. You can make a **pudding** with the nutrients of 2 cups fat-free milk, but the liquid of only 1¼ to 1½ cups by using ⅔ cup nonfat dry milk powder, a 4-serving package of sugar-free instant pudding, and the lesser amount of water. This makes the pudding taste much creamier and more like homemade. Also, pie filling made my way will set up in minutes. If company is knocking at your door, you can prepare a pie for them almost as fast as you can open the door and invite them in. And if by chance you have leftovers, the filling will not separate the way it does when you use the 2 cups of fat-free milk suggested on the package. (If you absolutely refuse to use this handy powdered milk, you can substitute

fat-free milk in the amount of water I call for. Your pie won't be as creamy, and will likely get runny if you have leftovers.)

2. You can make your own "**sour cream**" by combining ¾ cup plain fat-free yogurt with ⅓ cup nonfat dry milk powder. What you did by doing this is fourfold: (1) The dry milk stabilizes the yogurt and keeps the whey from separating. (2) The dry milk slightly helps to cut the tartness of the yogurt. (3) It's still virtually fat-free. (4) The calcium has been increased by 100 percent. Isn't it great how we can make that distant relative of sour cream a first kissin' cousin by adding the nonfat dry milk powder? Or, if you place 1 cup plain fat-free yogurt in a sieve lined with a coffee filter, and place the sieve over a small bowl and refrigerate for about 6 hours, you will end up with a very good alternative for sour cream. To **stabilize yogurt** when cooking or baking with it, just add 1 teaspoon cornstarch to every ¾ cup yogurt.

3. You can make **evaporated fat-free milk** by using ⅓ cup nonfat dry milk powder and ½ cup water for every ½ cup evaporated fat-free milk you need. This is handy to know when you want to prepare a recipe calling for evaporated fat-free milk and you don't have any in the cupboard. And if you are using a recipe that requires only 1 cup evaporated fat-free milk, you don't have to worry about what to do with the leftover milk in the can.

4. You can make **sugar-free and fat-free sweetened condensed milk** by using 1⅓ cups nonfat dry milk powder mixed with ½ cup cold water, microwaved on HIGH until the mixture is hot but not boiling. Then stir in ½ cup Splenda or pourable Sugar Twin. Cover and chill at least 4 hours.

5. For any recipe that calls for **buttermilk**, you might want to try **JO's Buttermilk**: Blend 1 cup water and ⅔ cup nonfat dry milk powder (the nutrients of 2 cups of fat-free milk). It'll be thicker than this mixed-up milk usually is, because it's doubled. Add 1 teaspoon white vinegar and stir, then let it sit for at least 10 minutes.

What else? Nonfat dry milk powder adds calcium without fuss to many recipes, and it can be stored for months in your refrigerator or freezer.

And for **a different taste when preparing sugar-free instant pudding mixes,** use ¾ cup plain fat-free yogurt for one of the required cups of milk. Blend as usual. It will be thicker and creamier—and no, it doesn't taste like yogurt.

Another **variation for the sugar-free instant vanilla pudding** is to use 1 cup fat-free milk and 1 cup crushed pineapple with juice. Mix as usual.

Soup Substitutes

One of my subscribers was looking for a way to further restrict salt intake and needed a substitute for **cream of mushroom soup.** For many of my recipes, I use Healthy Request Cream of Mushroom Soup, as it is a reduced-sodium product. The label suggests two servings per can, but I usually incorporate the soup into a recipe serving at least four. By doing this, I've reduced the sodium in the soup by half again.

But if you must restrict your sodium even more, try making my Healthy Exchanges **Creamy Mushroom Sauce.** Place 1½ cups evaporated fat-free milk and 3 tablespoons flour in a covered jar. Shake well and pour the mixture into a medium saucepan sprayed with butter-flavored cooking spray. Add ½ cup canned sliced mushrooms, rinsed and drained. Cook over medium heat, stirring often, until the mixture thickens. Add any seasonings of your choice. You can use this sauce in any recipe that calls for one 10¾-ounce can of cream of mushroom soup.

Why did I choose these proportions and ingredients?

- 1½ cups evaporated fat-free milk is the amount in one can.

- It's equal to three Fat-Free Milk choices or exchanges.

- It's the perfect amount of liquid and flour for a medium cream sauce.

- 3 tablespoons flour is equal to one Bread/Starch choice or exchange.

- Any leftovers will reheat beautifully with a flour-based sauce, but not with a cornstarch base.

- The mushrooms are one Vegetable choice or exchange.

- This sauce is virtually fat-free, sugar-free, and sodium-free.

Proteins

Eggs

I use eggs in moderation. I enjoy the real thing on an average of three to four times a week. So, my recipes are calculated on using whole eggs. However, if you choose to use egg substitute in place of the egg, the finished product will turn out just fine and the fat grams per serving will be even lower than those listed.

If you like the look, taste, and feel of **hard-boiled eggs** in salads but haven't been using them because of the cholesterol in the yolk, I have a couple of alternatives for you: (1) Pour an 8-ounce carton of egg substitute into a medium skillet sprayed with cooking spray. Cover the skillet tightly and cook over low heat until substitute is just set, about 10 minutes. Remove from heat and let set, still covered, for 10 minutes more. Uncover and cool completely. Chop the set mixture. This will make about 1 cup of chopped egg. (2) Even easier is to hard-boil "real eggs," toss the yolk away, and chop the white. Either way, you don't deprive yourself of the pleasure of egg in your salad.

In most recipes calling for **egg substitutes**, you can use 2 egg whites in place of the equivalent of 1 egg substitute. Just break the eggs open and toss the yolks away. I can hear some of you already saying, "But that's wasteful!" Well, take a look at the price on the egg substitute package (which usually has the equivalent of 4 eggs in it), then look at the price of a dozen eggs, from which you'd get the equivalent of 6 egg substitutes. Now, what's wasteful about that?

Meats

Whenever I include **cooked chicken** in a recipe, I use roasted white meat without skin. Whenever I include **roast beef** or **pork** in a recipe, I use the loin cuts because they are much leaner. However, most of the time I do my roasting of all these meats at the local deli. I just ask for a chunk of their lean roasted meat, 6 or 8 ounces, and ask them not to slice it. When I get home, I cube or dice the meat and am ready to use it in my recipe. The reason I do this is threefold: (1) I'm getting just the amount I need without leftovers; (2) I don't have the expense of heating the oven; and (3) I'm not throwing away the bone, gristle, and fat I'd be cutting off the meat. Overall, it is probably cheaper to "roast" it the way I do.

Did you know that you can make an acceptable meat loaf without using egg for the binding? Just replace every egg with ¼ cup of liquid. You could use beef broth, tomato sauce, even applesauce, to name just a few. For a meatloaf to serve 6, I always use 1 pound of extra-lean ground beef or turkey, 6 tablespoons of dried fine bread crumbs, and ¼ cup of the liquid, plus anything else healthy that strikes my fancy at the time. I mix well and place the mixture in an 8-by-8-inch baking dish or 9-by-5-inch loaf pan sprayed with cooking spray. Bake uncovered at 350 degrees for 35 to 50 minutes (depending on the added ingredients). You will never miss the egg.

Any time you are **browning ground meat** for a casserole and want to get rid of almost all the excess fat, just place the uncooked meat loosely in a plastic colander. Set the colander in a glass pie plate. Place in microwave and cook on HIGH for 3 to 6 minutes (depending on the amount being browned), stirring often. Use as you would for any casserole. You can also chop up onions and brown them with the meat if you want.

To **brown meat for any Italian dish** (and add some extra "zip"), simply pour a couple of tablespoons of fat-free Italian dressing into a skillet and add your ingredients to be browned. The dressing acts almost like olive oil in the process and adds a touch of flavor as well. And to make an **Italian Sloppy Joe**, brown 16 ounces extra-lean ground meat and 1 cup chopped onion in ¼ cup fat-free Italian dressing, then add 1 cup tomato sauce, lower heat, and simmer for 10 minutes. *Bravo!*

Remember, always opt for the leanest ground beef or turkey you can find. Here in DeWitt, we can buy 95% extra-lean ground sirloin, which provides about 8 to 10 grams fat in a 2 to 3 ounce serving. Lean ground turkey provides about 5 to 7 grams of fat. But cheaper cuts can "cost" you up to 20 grams of fat per serving. It's standard practice to grind the skin into inexpensive ground turkey found in most one-pound frozen packages, so beware.

Gravy and Mashed Potatoes

For **gravy** with all the "old time" flavor but without the extra fat, try this almost effortless way to prepare it. First, pour your pan drippings (from roasted turkey, roast beef, or roast pork) into a large cake pan and set the pan in your freezer for at least 15 to 20 minutes so that the fat can congeal on the top and be skimmed off. Use a large pan even if you only have a small amount of drippings so that you get maximum air exposure for quick congealing. (If you prefer, you can purchase one of those fat separator pitchers that separates the fat from the juice.)

Pour your defatted juice into a large skillet. This recipe begins with about one cup of "stock." Now, pour either one cup of potato water (water that potatoes were boiled in before mashing) or regular water into a large jar. Potato water is my first choice because it's loaded with nutrients so I use it whenever I'm making fresh mashed potatoes to go with my homemade gravy. Add 3 tablespoons of all-purpose flour, screw the lid on, and shake until the mixture is well-blended. This easy step assures that you won't get lumps in your gravy!

Pour the mixture into the skillet with defatted stock and add any seasonings you like. Cook over medium heat, stirring constantly with a wire whisk, until mixture thickens and starts to boil. (The whisk is another "secret" for lump-free gravy.) Now pour the gravy into your prettiest gravy bowl and serve with pride!

Why did I use flour instead of cornstarch? Because any left-overs will reheat nicely with the flour base and will not with a corn-starch base. Also, 3 tablespoons of flour works out to 1 Bread/Starch exchange. This virtually fat-free gravy makes about 2 cups, so you could spoon about ½ cup gravy on your low-fat mashed potatoes and only have to count your gravy as ¼ Bread/Starch exchange.

Here's how to make the **best mashed potatoes:** For a 6-serving batch, quarter 6 medium potatoes and boil until they are tender in just enough water to cover them. Drain the potatoes, but *do not* throw the water away. Return the potatoes to the saucepan, whip them gently with an electric mixer, then add about ½ cup of the reserved potato water, ⅓ cup Carnation nonfat dry milk powder, and 2 tablespoons fat-free sour cream. Continue whipping with the mixer until smooth. You're sure to be begged to share the "secret" of your creamy mashed potatoes!

Fruits and Vegetables

If you want to enjoy a **"fruit shake"** with some pizzazz, just combine soda water and unsweetened fruit juice in a blender. Add crushed ice. Blend on HIGH until thick. Refreshment without guilt.

You'll see that many recipes use ordinary **canned vegetables.** They're much cheaper than reduced-sodium versions, and once you rinse and drain them, the sodium is reduced anyway. I believe in saving money wherever possible so we can afford the best fat-free and sugar-free products as they come onto the market.

All three kinds of **vegetables—fresh, frozen, and canned—** have their place in a healthy diet. My husband, Cliff, hates the taste of frozen or fresh green beans, thinks the texture is all wrong, so I use canned green beans instead. In this case, canned vegetables have their proper place when I'm feeding my husband. If someone in your family has a similar concern, it's important to respond to it so everyone can be happy and enjoy the meal.

When I use **fruits or vegetables** like apples, cucumbers, and zucchini, I wash them really well and **leave the skin on.** It provides added color, fiber, and attractiveness to any dish. And, because I use processed flour in my cooking, I like to increase the fiber in my diet by eating my fruits and vegetables in their closest-to-natural state.

To help **keep fresh fruits and veggies fresh,** just give them a quick "shower" with lemon juice. The easiest way to do this is to pour purchased lemon juice into a kitchen spray bottle and store in the refrigerator. Then, every time you use fresh fruits or vegetables in a salad or dessert, simply give them a quick spray with your "lemon spritzer." You just might be amazed by how this little trick keeps your produce from turning brown so fast.

Another great way to **keep fruits from turning brown**: try dipping them in Diet Mountain Dew!

Here's a way to enjoy **cranberries** all year round: buy a few extra bags while they are in season and freeze them for future use. By the way, cranberries chop better when frozen!

The next time you warm canned vegetables such as carrots or green beans, drain and heat the vegetables in ¼ cup beef or chicken broth. It gives a nice variation to an old standby. Here's a simple **white sauce** for vegetables and casseroles without using added fat that can be made by spraying a medium saucepan with butter-flavored cooking spray. Place 1½ cups evaporated fat-free milk and 3 tablespoons flour in a covered jar. Shake well. Pour into the sprayed saucepan and cook over medium heat until thick, stirring constantly. Add salt and pepper to taste. You can also add ½ cup canned drained mushrooms and/or 3 ounces (¾ cup) shredded reduced-fat cheese. Continue cooking until the cheese melts.

Zip up canned or frozen green beans with **chunky salsa**: ½ cup to 2 cups beans. Heat thoroughly. Chunky salsa also makes a wonderful dressing on lettuce salads. It only counts as a vegetable, so enjoy.

Another wonderful **South of the Border dressing** can be

stirred up by using ½ cup of chunky salsa and ¼ cup fat-free ranch dressing. Cover and store in your refrigerator. Use as a dressing for salads or as a topping for baked potatoes.

To **"roast" green or red peppers,** pierce a whole pepper in four or six places with the tines of a fork, then place the pepper in a glass pie plate and microwave on HIGH for 10 to 12 minutes, turning after every 4 minutes. Cover and let set for 5 minutes. Then, remove the seeds and peel the skin off and cut into strips. Use right away or freeze for future use.

Delightful Dessert Ideas

For a special treat that tastes anything but "diet," try placing **spreadable fruit** in a container and microwave for about 15 seconds. Then pour the melted fruit spread over a serving of nonfat ice cream or frozen yogurt. One tablespoon of spreadable fruit is equal to 1 Fruit choice or exchange. Some combinations to get you started are apricot over chocolate ice cream, strawberry over strawberry ice cream, or any flavor over vanilla.

Another way I use spreadable fruit is to make a delicious **topping for a cheesecake or angel food cake.** I take ½ cup fruit and ½ cup Cool Whip Lite and blend the two together with a teaspoon of coconut extract.

Here's a really **good topping** for the fall of the year. Place 1½ cups unsweetened applesauce in a medium saucepan or 4-cup glass measure. Stir in 2 tablespoons raisins, 1 teaspoon apple pie spice, and 2 tablespoons Cary's Sugar Free Maple Syrup. Cook over medium heat on the stovetop or microwave on HIGH until warm. Then spoon about ½ cup of the warm mixture over pancakes, French toast, or sugar- and fat-free vanilla ice cream. It's as close as you will get to guilt-free apple pie!

Do you love hot fudge sundaes as much as I do? Here's my secret for making **Almost Sinless Hot Fudge Sauce.** Just combine the contents of a 4-serving package of Jell-O sugar-free chocolate cook-and-serve pudding with ⅔ cup Carnation Nonfat Dry Milk Powder in a medium saucepan. Add 1¼ cups water. Cook over medium heat, stirring constantly with a wire whisk, until the mixture thickens and starts to boil. Remove from heat and stir in 1 teaspoon vanilla extract, 2 teaspoons reduced-calorie margarine, and ½ cup miniature marshmallows. This makes six ¼ cup servings. Any leftovers can be refrigerated and reheated later in the microwave. Yes, you can buy fat-free chocolate syrup nowadays, but have you checked the sugar content? For a ¼-cup serving of store-bought syrup (and you show me any true hot fudge sundae lover who would settle for less than ¼ cup) it clocks in at over 150 calories with 39 grams of sugar! Hershey's Lite Syrup, while better, still has 100 calories and 10 grams of sugar. But this "homemade" version costs you only 60 calories, less than ½ gram of fat, and just 6 grams of sugar for the same ¼-cup serving. For an occasional squirt on something where 1 teaspoon is enough, I'll use Hershey's Lite Syrup. But when I crave a hot fudge sundae, I scoop out some sugar- and fat-free ice cream, then spoon my Almost Sinless Hot Fudge Sauce over the top and smile with pleasure.

A quick yet tasty way to prepare **strawberries for shortcake** is to place about ¾ cup sliced strawberries, 2 tablespoons Diet Mountain Dew, and sugar substitute to equal ¼ cup sugar in a blender container. Process on BLEND until mixture is smooth. Pour the mixture into bowl. Add 1¼ cups sliced strawberries and mix well. Cover and refrigerate until ready to serve with shortcakes. This tastes just like the strawberry sauce I remember my mother making when I was a child.

Here's a wonderful secret for **making shortcakes:** just follow the recipe for shortcakes on the Bisquick Reduced Fat Baking Mix box, but substitute Splenda or pourable Sugar Twin for the sugar, fat-free milk for the regular milk, and fat-free sour cream for the margarine. When you serve these light and tasty shortcakes to your loved ones, I defy any of them to notice the difference between your version and the original!

Have you tried **thawing Cool Whip Lite** by stirring it? Don't! You'll get a runny mess and ruin the look and taste of your dessert. You can *never* treat Cool Whip Lite the same way you did regular Cool Whip because the "lite" version just doesn't contain enough fat. Thaw your Cool Whip Lite by placing it in your refrigerator at least two hours before you need to use it. When they took the excess fat out of Cool Whip to make it "lite," they replaced it with air. When you stir the living daylights out of it to hurry up the thawing, you also stir out the air. You also can't thaw your Cool Whip Lite in the microwave, or you'll end up with Cool Whip Soup!

Always have a thawed container of Cool Whip Lite in your refrigerator, as it keeps well for up to two weeks. It actually freezes and thaws and freezes and thaws again quite well, so if you won't be using it soon, you could refreeze your leftovers. Just remember to take it out a few hours before you need it, so it'll be creamy and soft and ready to use.

Remember, anytime you see the words *fat-free* or *reduced-fat* on the labels of cream cheese, sour cream, or whipped topping, handle it gently. The fat has been replaced by air or water, and the product has to be treated with special care.

How can you **frost an entire pie with just ½ cup of whipped topping**? First, don't use an inexpensive brand. I use Cool Whip Lite or La Creme Lite. Make sure the topping is fully thawed. Always spread from the center to the sides using a rubber spatula. This way, ½ cup topping will cover an entire pie. Remember, the operative word is *frost,* not pile the entire container on top of the pie!

Here's my vote for the easiest **crumb topping** ever! Simply combine 3 tablespoons of purchased graham cracker crumbs (or three 2½-inch squares made into fine crumbs) with 2 teaspoons reduced-calorie margarine and 1 tablespoon (if desired) chopped nuts. Mix this well and sprinkle evenly over the top of your fruit pie and bake as you normally would. You can use either a purchased graham cracker piecrust or an unbaked refrigerated regular piecrust. Another almost effortless crumb topping can be made by combining 6 tablespoons Bisquick Reduced Fat Baking Mix and 2 tablespoons Splenda or pourable Sugar Twin with 2 teaspoons of reduced-calorie margarine until the mixture becomes crumbly. Again, you can stir in 1 tablespoon of chopped nuts if you wish. Evenly sprinkle this mixture over your fruit filling and bake as usual. This works best with a purchased unbaked refrigerated pie crust.

Another trick I often use is to include tiny amounts of "real people" food, such as coconut, but **extend the flavor by using extracts**. Try it—you will be surprised by how little of the real thing you can use and still feel you are not being deprived.

If you are preparing a pie filling that has ample moisture, just line the bottom of a 9-by-9-inch cake pan with **graham crackers.** Pour the filling over the top of the crackers. Cover and refrigerate until the moisture has enough time to soften the crackers. Overnight is best. This eliminates the added **fats and sugars of a piecrust.**

One of my readers provided a smart and easy way to enjoy a **two-crust pie** without all the fat that usually comes along with those two crusts. Just use one Pillsbury refrigerated piecrust. Let it set at room temperature for about 20 minutes. Cut the crust in half on the folded line. Gently roll each half into a ball. Wipe your counter with a wet cloth and place a sheet of wax paper on it. Put one of the balls on the wax paper, then cover with another piece of wax paper, and roll it out with your rolling pin. Carefully remove the wax paper on one side and place that side into your 8- or 9-inch pie plate. Fill with your usual pie filling, then repeat the process for the top crust. Bake as usual. Enjoy!

Here's a good tip for **avoiding a "doughy" taste when using a refrigerated piecrust.** Make sure you take the piecrust out of the refrigerator and let it sit on the counter for at least 10 minutes before putting it in the pie plate and baking it. If you put the piecrust into the plate before it has a chance to "warm up," it will be stiffer than if you let it come to room temperature before using. This means that the tiny amount of flour clinging to the crust doesn't have a chance to become "one" with the crust, making the finished product "doughier."

When you are preparing a pie that uses a purchased piecrust, simply tear out the paper label on the plastic cover (but do check it for a coupon good on a future purchase) and turn the cover upside-down over the prepared pie. You now have a cover that protects your beautifully garnished pie from having anything fall on top of it. It makes the pie very portable when it's your turn to bring dessert to a get-together.

And for **"picture-perfect" presentation** when using a purchased piecrust, just remove the protective plastic cover, place a pizza pan over the top of the crust, invert the "tin pan" and carefully remove it so the bottom of the crust is exposed. Then, replace the "tin pan" with an attractive pottery pie plate and, with one hand holding each pan in place, flip the piecrust so that the piecrust is now sitting securely in the pottery plate. Remove the pizza pan and fill with your favorite Healthy Exchanges pie filling. This is easier than it sounds, and it makes your dessert look extra-special!

Did you know you can make your own **fruit-flavored yogurt**? Mix 1 tablespoon of any flavor of spreadable fruit spread with ¾ cup plain yogurt. It's every bit as tasty and much cheaper. You can also make your own **lemon yogurt** by combining 3 cups plain fat-free yogurt with 1 tub Crystal Light lemonade powder. Mix well, cover, and store in the refrigerator. I think you will be pleasantly surprised by the ease, cost, and flavor of this "made from scratch" calcium-rich treat. P.S.: You can make any flavor you like by using any of the Crystal Light mixes—Cranberry? Iced Tea? You decide.

Other Smart Substitutions

Many people have inquired about **substituting applesauce and artificial sweetener for butter and sugar,** but what if you aren't satisfied with the result? One woman wrote to me about a recipe for her grandmother's cookies that called for 1 cup of butter and 1½ cups of sugar. Well, any recipe that depends on as much butter and sugar as this one does is generally not a good candidate for "healthy exchanges." The original recipe needed a large quantity of fat to produce a crisp cookie just like Grandma made.

Applesauce can often be used instead of vegetable oil but generally doesn't work well as a replacement for butter, margarine, or lard. If a recipe calls for ½ cup of vegetable oil or less and your recipe is for a bar cookie, quick bread, muffin, or cake mix, you can try substituting an equal amount of unsweetened applesauce. If the recipe calls for more, try using ½ cup applesauce and the rest oil. You're cutting down the fat but shouldn't end up with a taste disaster! This "applesauce shortening" works great in many recipes, but so far I haven't been able to figure out a way to deep-fat fry with it!

Another rule for healthy substitution: Up to ½ cup sugar or less can be replaced by *an artificial sweetener that can withstand the heat of baking,* like pourable Sugar Twin or Splenda. If it requires more than ½ cup sugar, cut the amount needed by 75 percent and use ½ cup sugar substitute and sugar for the rest. Other options: reduce the butter and sugar by 25 percent and see if the finished product still satisfies you in taste and appearance. Or, make the cookies just like Grandma did, realizing they are part of your family's holiday tradition. Enjoy a *moderate* serving of a couple of cookies once or twice during the season, and just forget about them the rest of the year.

Did you know that you can replace the fat in many quick breads, muffins, and shortcakes with **fat-free mayonnaise** or **fat-free sour cream**? This can work if the original recipe doesn't call for a lot of fat *and* sugar. If the recipe is truly fat and sugar dependent, such as traditional sugar cookies, cupcakes, or pastries, it won't work. Those recipes require the large amounts of sugar and fat to make love in the dark of the oven to produce a tender finished product. But if you have a favorite quick bread that doesn't call for a lot of sugar or fat, why don't you give one of these substitutes a try?

If you enjoy beverage mixes like those from Alba, here are my Healthy Exchanges versions:

For **chocolate flavored,** use ⅓ cup nonfat dry milk powder and 2 tablespoons Nestlé Sugar-Free Chocolate Flavored Quik. Mix well and use as usual. Or, use ⅓ cup nonfat dry milk powder, 1 teaspoon unsweetened cocoa, and sugar substitute to equal 3 tablespoons sugar. Mix well and use as usual.

For **vanilla flavored**, use ⅓ cup nonfat dry milk powder, sugar substitute to equal 2 tablespoons sugar, and add 1 teaspoon vanilla extract when adding liquid.

For **strawberry flavored**, use ⅓ cup nonfat dry milk powder, sugar substitute to equal 2 tablespoons sugar, and add 1 teaspoon strawberry extract and 3–4 drops red food coloring when adding liquid.

Each of these makes one packet of drink mix. If you need to double the recipe, double everything but the extract. Use 1½ teaspoons of extract or it will be too strong. Use 1 cup cold water with one recipe mix to make a glass of flavored milk. If you want to make a shake, combine the mix, water, and 3–4 ice cubes in your blender, then process on BLEND till smooth.

A handy tip when making **healthy punch** for a party: Prepare a few extra cups of your chosen drink, freeze it in cubes in a couple of ice trays, then keep your punch from "watering down" by cooling it with punch cubes instead of ice cubes.

What should you do if you can't find the product listed in a Healthy Exchanges recipe? You can substitute in some cases—use Lemon Jell-O if you can't find Hawaiian Pineapple, for example. But if you're determined to track down the product you need, and your own store manager hasn't been able to order it for you, why not use one of the new online grocers and order exactly what you need, no matter where you live. Try **http://www.netgrocer.com**.

Not all low-fat cooking products are interchangeable, as one of my readers recently discovered when she tried to cook pancakes on her griddle using I Can't Believe It's Not Butter! spray—and they stuck! This butter-flavored spray is wonderful for a quick squirt on air-popped popcorn or corn on the cob, and it's great for topping your pancakes once they're cooked. In fact, my taste buds have to check twice because it tastes so much like real butter! (And this is high praise from someone who once thought butter was the most perfect food ever created.)

But I Can't Believe It's Not Butter! doesn't work well for sautéing or browning. After trying to fry an egg with it and cooking up a disaster, I knew this product had its limitations. So I decided to continue using Pam or Weight Watchers butter-flavored cooking spray whenever I'm browning anything in a skillet or on a griddle.

Many of my readers have reported difficulty finding a product I use in many recipes: Jell-O cook-and-serve pudding. I have three suggestions for those of you with this problem:

1. **Work with your grocery store manager to get this product into your store,** and then make sure you and everyone you know buys it by the bagful! Products that sell well are reordered and kept in stock, especially with today's computerized cash registers that record what's purchased. You may also want to write or call Kraft General Foods and ask for their help. They can be reached at (800) 431-1001 weekdays from 9 A.M. to 4 P.M. (EST).

2. **You can prepare a recipe that calls for cook-and-serve pudding by using instant pudding of the same flavor.** Yes, that's right, you **can** cook with the instant when making my recipes. The finished product won't be quite as wonderful, but still at least a 3 on a 4-star scale. You can never do the opposite—never use cook-and-serve in a recipe that calls for instant! One time at a cooking demonstration, I could not understand why my Blueberry Mountain Cheesecake never did set up. Then I spotted the box in the trash and noticed I'd picked the wrong type of pudding mix. Be careful—the boxes are both blue, but the instant has pudding on a silver spoon, and the cook-and-serve has a stream of milk running down the front into a bowl with a wooden spoon.

3. **You can make JO's Sugar-Free Vanilla Cook-and-Serve Pudding Mix instead of using Jell-O's.** Here's my recipe: 2 tablespoons cornstarch, ½ cup pourable Sugar Twin or Splenda, ⅔ cup Carnation Nonfat Dry Milk Powder, 1½ cups water, 2 teaspoons vanilla extract, and 4 to 5 drops yellow food coloring. Combine all this in a medium saucepan and cook over medium heat, stirring constantly, until the mixture comes to a full boil and thickens. This is for basic cooked vanilla sugar-free pudding. For a chocolate version, the recipe is 2 tablespoons cornstarch, ¼ cup pourable Sugar Twin or Splenda, 2 tablespoons sugar-free chocolate-flavored Nestle's Quik, 1½ cups water, and 1 teaspoon vanilla extract. Follow the same cooking instructions as for the vanilla.

If you're preparing this as part of a recipe that also calls for adding a package of gelatin, just stir that into the mix.

Adapting a favorite family cake recipe? Here's something to try: replace an egg and oil in the original with ⅓ cup fat-free yogurt and ¼ cup fat-free mayonnaise. Blend these two ingredients with your liquids in a separate bowl, then add the yogurt mixture to the flour mixture and mix gently just to combine. (You don't want to overmix or you'll release the gluten in the batter and end up with a tough batter.)

Want a tasty coffee creamer without all the fat? You could use Carnation's Fat Free Coffeemate, which is 10 calories per teaspoon, but if you drink several cups a day with several teaspoons each, that adds up quickly to nearly 100 calories a day! Why not try my version? It's not quite as creamy, but it is good. Simply combine ⅓ cup Carnation Nonfat Dry Milk Powder and ¼ cup Splenda or pourable Sugar Twin. Cover and store in your cupboard or refrigerator. At 3 calories per teaspoon, you can enjoy three teaspoons for less than the calories of one teaspoon of the purchased variety.

Some Helpful Hints

Sugar-free puddings and gelatins are important to many of my recipes, but if you prefer to avoid sugar substitutes, you could still prepare the recipes with regular puddings or gelatins. The calories would be higher, but you would still be cooking low-fat.

When a recipe calls for **chopped nuts** (and you only have whole ones), who wants to dirty the food processor just for a couple of tablespoonsful? You could try to chop them using your cutting board, but be prepared for bits and pieces to fly all over the kitchen. I use "Grandma's food processor." I take the biggest nuts I can find, put them in a small glass bowl, and chop them into chunks just the right size using a metal biscuit cutter.

To quickly **toast nuts** without any fuss, spread about ½ cup of nuts (any kind) in a glass pie plate and microwave on HIGH (100% power) for 6 to 7 minutes or until golden. Stir after the first 3 minutes, then after each minute until done. Store them in an airtight container in your refrigerator. Toasting nuts really brings out their flavor, so it seems as if you used a whole treeful instead of tiny amounts.

A quick hint about **reduced-fat peanut butter:** don't store it in the refrigerator. Because the fat has been reduced, it won't spread as easily when it's cold. Keep it in your cupboard and a little will spread a lot further.

Crushing **graham crackers** for topping? A self-seal sandwich bag works great!

An eleven-year-old fan e-mailed me with a great tip recently: if you can't find the **mini chocolate chips** I use in many recipes, simply purchase the regular size and put them in a nut grinder to coarsely chop them.

If you have a **leftover muffin** and are looking for something a little different for breakfast, you can make **a "breakfast sundae."** Crumble the muffin into a cereal bowl. Sprinkle a serving of fresh fruit over it and top with a couple of tablespoons of plain fat-free yogurt sweetened with sugar substitute and your choice of extract. The thought of it just might make you jump out of bed with a smile on your face. (Speaking of muffins, did you know that if you fill the unused muffin wells with water when baking muffins, you help ensure more even baking and protect the muffin pan at the same time?) Another muffin hint: lightly spray the inside of paper baking cups with butter-flavored cooking spray before spooning the muffin batter into them. Then you won't end up with paper clinging to your fresh-baked muffins.

The secret of making **good meringues** without sugar is to use 1 tablespoon of Splenda or pourable Sugar Twin for every egg white, and a small amount of extract. Use ½ to 1 teaspoon for the batch. Almond, vanilla, and coconut are all good choices. Use the same amount of cream of tartar you usually do. Bake the meringue in the same old way. Even if you can't eat sugar, you can enjoy a healthy meringue pie when it's prepared *The Healthy Exchanges Way.* (Remember that egg whites whip up best at room temperature.)

Try **storing your Bisquick Reduced Fat Baking Mix** in the freezer. It won't freeze, and it *will* stay fresh much longer. (It works for coffee, doesn't it?)

To check if your **baking powder** is fresh, put 1 teaspoonful in a bowl and pour 2 tablespoons of very hot tap water over it. If it's fresh, it will bubble very actively. If it doesn't bubble, then it's time to replace your old can with a new one.

If you've ever wondered about **changing ingredients** in one of my recipes, the answer is that some things can be changed to suit your family's tastes, but others should not be tampered with. **Don't change**: the amount of flour, bread crumbs, reduced-fat baking mix, baking soda, baking powder, or liquid or dry milk powder. And if I include a small amount of salt, it's necessary for the recipe to turn out correctly. **What you can change:** an extract flavor (if you don't like coconut, choose vanilla or almond instead); a spreadable fruit flavor; the type of fruit in a pie filling (but be careful about substituting fresh for frozen and vice versa—sometimes it works, but it may not); the flavor of pudding or gelatin. As long as package sizes and amounts are the same, go for it. It will never hurt my feelings if you change a recipe, so please your family—don't worry about me!

Because I always say that "good enough" isn't good enough for me anymore, here's a way to make your cup of **fat-free and sugar-free hot cocoa** more special. After combining the hot chocolate mix and hot water, stir in ½ teaspoon vanilla extract and a light sprinkle of cinnamon. If you really want to feel decadent, add a tablespoon of Cool Whip Lite. Isn't life grand?

If you must limit your sugar intake, but you love the idea of sprinkling **powdered sugar** on dessert crepes or burritos, here's a pretty good substitute: Place 1 cup Splenda or pourable Sugar Twin and 1 teaspoon cornstarch in a blender container, then cover and process on HIGH until the mixture resembles powdered sugar in texture, about 45 to 60 seconds. Store in an airtight container and use whenever you want a dusting of "powdered sugar" on any dessert.

Want my "almost instant" pies to set up even more quickly? Do as one of my readers does: freeze your Keebler piecrusts. Then, when you stir up one of my pies and pour the filling into the frozen crust, it sets up within seconds.

Some of my "island-inspired" recipes call for **rum or brandy extracts,** which provide the "essence" of liquor without the real thing. I'm a teetotaler by choice, so I choose not to include real liquor in any of my recipes. They're cheaper than liquor and you won't feel the need to shoo your kids away from the goodies. If you prefer not to use liquor extracts in your cooking, you can always substitute vanilla extract.

Did you know you can make your own single-serving bags of microwave popcorn? Spoon 2 tablespoons of popping kernels into a paper lunch bag, folding the top over twice to seal and placing the sealed bag in the microwave. Microwave on HIGH for 2 to 3 minutes, or until the popping stops. Then pour the popcorn into a large bowl and lightly spritz with I Can't Believe It's Not Butter! spray. You'll have 3 cups of virtually fat-free popcorn to munch on at a fraction of the price of purchased microwave popcorn.

Some Healthy Cooking Challenges and How I Solved 'Em

When you stir up one of my pie fillings, do you ever have a problem with **lumps?** Here's an easy solution for all of you "careful" cooks out there. Lumps occur when the pudding starts to set up before you can get the dry milk powder incorporated into the mixture. I always advise you to dump, pour, and stir fast with that wire whisk, letting no more than 30 seconds elapse from beginning to end.

But if you are still having problems, you can always combine the dry milk powder and the water in a separate bowl before adding the pudding mix and whisking quickly. Why don't I suggest this right from the beginning? Because that would mean an extra dish to wash every time—and you know I hate to wash dishes!

With a little practice and a light touch, you should soon get the hang of my original method. But now you've got an alternative way to lose those lumps!

I love the chemistry of foods, and so I've gotten great pleasure from analyzing what makes fat-free products tick. By dissecting these "miracle" products, I've learned how to make them work best. They require different handling than the high-fat products we're used to, but if treated properly, these slimmed-down versions can produce delicious results!

Fat-free sour cream: This product is wonderful on a hot baked potato, but have you noticed that it tends to be much gummier than regular sour cream? If you want to use it in a stroganoff dish or baked product, you must stir a tablespoon or two of fat-free milk into the fat-free sour cream before adding it to other ingredients.

Cool Whip Free: When the fat went out of the formula, air was stirred in to fill the void. So, if you stir it too vigorously, you release the air and *decrease* the volume. Handle it with kid gloves—gently. Since the manufacturer forgot to ask for my input, I'll share with you how to make it taste almost the same as it used to. Let the container thaw in the refrigerator, then ever so gently stir in 1 teaspoon vanilla extract. Now, put the lid back on and enjoy it a tablespoon at a time, the same way you did Cool Whip Lite.

Fat-free cream cheese: When the fat was removed from this product, water replaced it. So don't ever use an electric mixer on the fat-free version or you risk releasing the water and having your finished product look more like dip than cheesecake! Stirring it gently with a sturdy spoon in a glass bowl with a handle will soften it just as much as it needs to be. (A glass bowl with a handle lets you see what's going on; the handle gives you control as you stir. This "user-friendly" method is good for tired cooks, young cooks, and cooks with arthritis!) And don't be alarmed if the cream cheese gets caught in your wire whisk when you start combining the pudding mix and other ingredients. Just keep knocking it back down into the bowl by hitting the whisk against the rim of the bowl, and as you continue blending, it will soften even more and drop off the whisk. When it's time to pour the filling into your crust, your whisk shouldn't have anything much clinging to it.

Reduced-fat margarine: Again, the fat was replaced by water. If you try to use the reduced-fat kind in your cookie recipe spoon for spoon, you will end up with a cakelike cookie instead of the crisp kind most of us enjoy. You have to take into consideration that some water will be released as the product bakes. Use less liquid than the recipe calls for (when re-creating family recipes *only*—I've figured that into Healthy Exchanges recipes). And never, never, never use fat-*free* margarine and expect anyone to ask for seconds!

When every minute counts, and you need 2 cups cooked noodles for a casserole, how do you **figure out how much of a box of pasta to prepare?** Here's a handy guide that should help. While your final amount might vary slightly because of how loosely or tightly you "stuff" your measuring cup, this will make life easier.

Type	Start with this amount uncooked	If you want this amount cooked
Noodles	1 cup	1 cup
(thin, medium,	1¼ cups	1½ cups
wide, and mini	1¾ cups	2 cups
lasagne)	2¼ cups	2½ cups
	2½ cups	3 cups
Macaroni	⅓ cup	½ cup
(medium shells	⅔ cup	1 cup
and elbow)	1 cup	1½ cups
	1⅓ cups	2 cups
	2 cups	3 cups
Spaghetti,	¾ cup	1 cup
fettuccine,	1 cup	1½ cups
and rotini	1½ cups	2 cups
pasta	2½ cups	3 cups
Rice (instant)	⅓ cup	½ cup
	⅔ cup	1 cup

Type	Start with this amount uncooked	If you want this amount cooked
Rice (instant) (continued)	1 cup	1½ cups
	1⅓ cups	2 cups
	2 cups	3 cups
Rice (regular)	¼ cup	½ cup
	½ cup	1 cup
	1 cup	2 cups
	1½ cups	3 cups

Here's a handy idea for **keeping your cookbooks open** to a certain page while cooking: use two rubber bands, one wrapped vertically around the left side of the book, another on the right side. And to **keep your cookbooks clean**, try slipping the rubber-banded book into a gallon-sized Ziploc bag. (Though I'd consider it a compliment to know that the pages of my cookbooks were all splattered, because it would mean that you are really using the recipes!)

Homemade or Store-Bought?

I've been asked which is better for you: homemade from scratch, or purchased foods. My answer is *both!* Each has a place in a healthy lifestyle, and what that place is has everything to do with you.

Take **piecrusts,** for instance. If you love spending your spare time in the kitchen preparing foods, and you're using low-fat, low-sugar, and reasonably low sodium ingredients, go for it! But if, like so many people, your time is limited and you've learned to read labels, you could be better off using purchased foods.

I know that when I prepare a pie (and I experiment with a couple of pies each week, because this is Cliff's favorite dessert), I use a purchased crust. Why? Mainly because I can't make a good-tasting piecrust that is lower in fat than the brands I use. Also, purchased piecrusts fit my rule of "If it takes longer to fix than to eat, forget it!"

I've checked the nutrient information for the purchased piecrusts against recipes for traditional and "diet" piecrusts, using my computer software program. The purchased crust calculated lower in both fat and calories! I have tried some low-fat and low-sugar recipes, but they just didn't spark my taste buds, or were so complicated you needed an engineering degree just to get the crust in the pie plate.

I'm very happy with the purchased piecrusts in my recipes, because the finished product rarely, if ever, has more than 30 percent of total calories coming from fats. I also believe that we have to prepare foods our families and friends will eat with us on a regular basis and not feel deprived, or we've wasted time, energy, and money.

I could use a purchased "lite" **pie filling,** but instead I make my own. Here I can save both fat and sugar, and still make the filling almost as fast as opening a can. The bottom line: know what you have to spend when it comes to both time and fat/sugar calories, then make the best decision you can for you and your family. And don't go without an occasional piece of pie because you think it isn't *necessary*. A delicious pie prepared in a healthy way is one of the simple pleasures of life. It's a little thing, but it can make all the difference between just getting by with the bare minimum and living a full and healthy lifestyle.

I'm sure you'll add to this list of cooking tips as you begin preparing Healthy Exchanges recipes and discover how easy it can be to adapt your own favorite recipes using these ideas and your own common sense.

Planning Your "On the Go" Cooking Needs Before Leaving Home

Just as you consult a map before motoring out of your driveway, it's wise to do a little food pre-planning before you leave home. Also, it's a good idea to keep a running list of your inventory; when you use something, make a note of it. This makes your life much easier when you stop at a grocery store to restock your supplies. (I'm not listing salt and pepper, plastic tableware, and stainless steel flatware in the list—I know you'll remember to pack those!)

- Canned vegetables
- Canned meats, poultry, and fish
- Canned applesauce
- Canned fruits
- Canned bacon bits and tomato sauce
- Macaroni, spaghetti, and noodles
- Instant rice
- Graham crackers
- Sugar-free instant puddings
- Sugar-free instant gelatins

- Purchased piecrusts
- Peanut butter
- Fruit spread
- Reduced-fat and reduced-sodium soups
- Canned chicken and beef broth
- Soda crackers
- Evaporated fat-free milk
- Nonfat dry milk powder
- Salsa
- Ketchup
- Mustard
- Pickle relish
- Pickles
- Fat-free mayonnaise
- Worcestershire sauce
- Lemon juice
- Vinegar
- Fat-free dressings
- Cooking spray
- Flour
- Sugar substitutes
- Spices

A Peek into
My Pantry and
My Favorite Brands

Everyone asks me what foods I keep on hand and what brands I use. There are lots of good products on the grocery shelves today—many more than we dreamed about even a year or two ago. And I can't wait to see what's out there twelve months from now. The following are my staples and, where appropriate, my favorites *at this time*. I feel that these products are healthier, tastier, easy to get—and deliver the most flavor for the least amount of fat, sugar, or calories. If you find others you like as well *or better*, please use them. This is only a guide to make your grocery shopping and cooking easier. ***Following this list, you'll find my list of non-perishable ingredients that make cooking on the go a pleasure!

> *Fat-free plain yogurt* (Dannon)
> *Nonfat dry milk powder* (Carnation)
> *Evaporated fat-free milk* (Carnation)
> *Fat-free milk*
> *Fat-free cottage cheese*
> *Fat-free cream cheese* (Philadelphia)
> *Fat-free mayonnaise* (Kraft)
> *Fat-free salad dressings* (Kraft and Hendrickson's)
> *No-fat sour cream* (Land O Lakes)
> *Reduced-calorie margarine* (I Can't Believe It's Not Butter! Light)
> *Cooking sprays*
>   *Olive oil–flavored* (Pam)
>   *Butter-flavored* (Pam)
>   *Butter-flavored for spritzing* after *cooking* (I Can't Believe It's
>   Not Butter!)

Cooking oil (Puritan canola oil)
Reduced-calorie whipped topping (Cool Whip Lite or Cool Whip
    Free)
Sugar substitute:
    White sugar substitute (Splenda)
    Brown sugar substitute (Brown Sugar Twin)
Sugar-free gelatin and pudding mixes (JELL-O)
Baking mix (Bisquick Reduced Fat)
Pancake mix (Aunt Jemima Reduced Calorie)
Sugar-free pancake syrup (Log Cabin or Cary's)
Parmesan cheese (Kraft Reduced Fat Parmesan Style Grated
    Topping)
Reduced-fat cheese (shredded and sliced) (Kraft 2% Reduced Fat)
Shredded frozen potatoes (Mr. Dell's or Ore Ida)
Spreadable fruit spread (Welch's or Smucker's)
Peanut butter (Peter Pan reduced-fat, Jif reduced-fat, or Skippy
    reduced-fat)
Chicken broth (Healthy Request)
Beef broth (Swanson)
Tomato sauce (Hunt's)
Canned soups (Healthy Request)
Reduced sodium tomato juice
Reduced sodium ketchup
Piecrust
    Unbaked (Pillsbury—in dairy case)
    Graham cracker, shortbread, and chocolate (Keebler)
Crescent rolls (Pillsbury Reduced Fat)
Pastrami and corned beef (Carl Buddig Lean)
Luncheon meats (Healthy Choice or Oscar Mayer)
Ham (Dubuque 97% fat-free and reduced-sodium or Healthy
    Choice)
Bacon bits (Hormel or Oscar Mayer)
Kielbasa sausage and frankfurters (Healthy Choice or Oscar
    Mayer Light)
Canned white chicken, packed in water (Swanson)
Canned tuna, packed in water (Starkist)
95 to 97 percent ground sirloin beef or turkey breast
Soda crackers (Nabisco Fat Free and Ritz Reduced Fat)
Reduced-calorie bread—40 calories per slice or less
Small hamburger buns—80 calories per bun
Rice—instant, regular, brown, and wild (Minute Rice)
Instant potato flakes

Noodles, spaghetti, macaroni, and rotini pasta
Salsa
Pickle relish—dill, sweet, and hot dog
Mustard—Dijon, prepared yellow, and spicy
Unsweetened apple and orange juice
Reduced-calorie cranberry juice cocktail (Ocean Spray)
Unsweetened applesauce (Musselman's)
Fruit—fresh, frozen (no sugar added), and canned in juice
Pie filling (Lucky Leaf No Sugar Added Cherry and Apple)
Spices—JO's Spices or any national brand
Vinegar—cider and distilled white
*Lemon and lime juice (in small plastic fruit-shaped bottles found in
    the produce section)*
Instant fruit beverage mixes (Crystal Light)
Sugar-free hot chocolate beverage mixes (Swiss Miss or Nesquik)
Sugar-free and fat-free ice cream (Wells Blue Bunny)

The items on my shopping list are everyday foods found in just about any grocery store in America. But all are as low in fat, sugar, calories, and sodium as I can find—and still taste good! I can make any recipe in my cookbooks and newsletters as long as I have my cupboards and refrigerator stocked with these items. Whenever I use the last of any one item, I just make sure I pick up another supply the next time I'm at the store.

If your grocer does not stock these items, why not ask if they can be ordered on a trial basis? If the store agrees to do so, be sure to tell your friends to stop by, so that sales are good enough to warrant restocking the new products. Competition for shelf space is fierce, so only products that sell well stay around.

The Healthy Exchanges® "On the Go" Kitchen

When I first started creating Healthy Exchanges recipes, I had a tiny galley kitchen with room for only one person. But it never stopped me from feeling the sky was the limit when it came to seeking out great healthy taste! Even though I have a bigger home kitchen now, what I learned in those early days was a real help when I started cooking on the go. The best advice I can give you is: don't waste space on equipment you don't really need. Here's a list of what I consider worth having. You can probably find most of what you need at a local discount store or garage sale. You'll find you can prepare healthy, quick, and delicious food with just the "basics."

Kitchen Equipment Recommendations

Good-quality nonstick skillet (10-inch with a lid)
Good-quality nonstick saucepans (small, medium, large, with lids)—If you choose Teflon-coated pans and skillets, your cleanup time will be greatly reduced.
An electric skillet is a nice addition.
8-by-8-inch baking dish

Disposable aluminum 9-by-9-inch baking pans

Rimmed cookie sheet (make sure it fits into YOUR oven with room to spare)

Heavy duty plastic set of 3 mixing bowls (the kind that nest inside each other)

Empty Cool Whip Lite containers and lids for refrigerator food storage

Plastic liquid measuring cups (1-cup and 4-cup)

Sharp knives (paring and butcher)

Cutting board

Rubber spatulas

Wire whisk

Measuring spoons

Dry measuring cups

Large slotted spoon

Tea kettle

Vegetable parer

Wire racks

Covered jar

Kitchen timer

Can opener

You're stocked, you're set—let's go!

The Recipes

How to Read a Healthy Exchanges® Recipe

The Healthy Exchanges Nutritional Analysis

Before using these recipes, you may wish to consult your physician or health-care provider to be sure they are appropriate for you. The information in this book is not intended to take the place of any medical advice. It reflects my experiences, studies, research, and opinions regarding healthy eating.

Each recipe includes nutritional information calculated in three ways:

Healthy Exchanges Weight Loss Choices™ or Exchanges
Calories; Fat, Protein, Carbohydrates, and Fiber in grams;
    Sodium and Calcium in milligrams
DIABETIC EXCHANGES

In every Healthy Exchanges recipe, the DIABETIC EXCHANGES have been calculated by a registered dietitian. All the other calculations were done by computer, using the Food Processor II software. When the ingredient listing gives more than one choice, the first ingredient listed is the one used in the recipe analysis. Due to inevitable variations in the ingredients you choose to use, the nutritional values should be considered approximate.

The annotation "(limited)" following Protein counts in some

recipes indicates that consumption of whole eggs should be limited to four per week.

Please note the following symbols:

☆ This star means read the recipe's directions carefully for special instructions about **division** of ingredients.

❋ This symbol indicates **FREEZES WELL.**

Easy Breakfast Dishes

I've been a morning person all my life, and when I'm home in DeWitt, I'm often up before the sun. I love the peace and quiet of those early mornings before the sun comes up, when the house is quiet and the day is all in front of me. It's not all that different when Cliff and I are on the road together. He likes to drive when the highway is less crowded, so we often head out before sunrise. (It's a habit that began when he was a long-distance trucker, driving coast-to-coast week in and week out.) But whether we're due for a long day in the motor home, or taking the car on a shorter trip, breakfast is an important meal for us. Eating something hearty and satisfying first thing in the morning sets a positive tone for the day.

I've given you an abundance of choices to start your day with good health and good taste. If your preference is for pancakes, you've got to try my **Blueberry Pancakes with Maple Banana Sauce;** if you always choose French toast for breakfast or brunch, I just know you'll smile when you taste my **Sour Cream French Toast;** and if you can't start your day without eggs and bacon, ham, or sausage, you've got some great choices, especially my **Morning Mix Up** and **Ham Scrambled Eggs Benedict.** Whatever you choose, you'll be fueled and ready for anything the day brings!

Easy Breakfast Dishes

Tropical Morning Oats

You might think I created this recipe on a steamy Southern morning as we drove to an early-morning radio appearance, but in fact I thought of it on a frosty cold day, when the flavors of the tropics held the promise that summer wasn't too far off! ☻ Serves 6

2 cups water
1 (12-fluid-ounce) can Carnation Evaporated Fat Free Milk
1 cup (3 ounces) quick oats
¼ cup Splenda Granular
2 tablespoons raisins
1 cup (1 medium) diced banana
2 tablespoons chopped pecans
2 tablespoons flaked coconut

In a medium saucepan, combine water, evaporated milk, and oats. Bring mixture to a boil. Lower heat, cover, and simmer for 5 minutes, stirring occasionally. Remove from heat. Add Splenda, raisins, banana, and pecans. Mix gently to combine. For each serving, spoon about ¾ cup mixture into a bowl and top with 1 teaspoon coconut.

Each serving equals:

HE: ⅔ Bread • ½ Fat-Free Milk • ½ Fruit • ⅓ Fat •
9 Optional Calories

163 Calories • 3 gm Fat • 8 gm Protein •
26 gm Carbohydrate • 84 mg Sodium •
173 mg Calcium • 2 gm Fiber

DIABETIC EXCHANGES: 1 Starch/Carbohydrate •
½ Fat-Free Milk • ½ Fruit

Yummy Cinnamon Breakfast Squares

You might hear a banging on the door of your RV when you start the day with these mmm-good pastry treats! It's the sweet scent of cinnamon and fresh-baked rolls that's sure to bring everyone running for a taste.   ☻   Serves 16 (2 each)

> 1 (8-ounce) can Pillsbury Reduced Fat Crescent Rolls
> ⅓ cup Splenda Granular
> 1 teaspoon ground cinnamon

Preheat oven to 375 degrees. Spray a rimmed 10-by-15-inch baking sheet with butter-flavored cooking spray. Unroll crescent rolls and pat into a sheet, being sure to seal perforations. In a small bowl, combine Splenda and cinnamon. Lightly spray top of rolls with butter-flavored cooking spray. Evenly sprinkle cinnamon mixture over top. Lightly spray top again with butter-flavored cooking spray. Bake for 5 to 7 minutes. Cut into 32 pieces.

Each serving equals:

HE: ½ Bread • 3 Optional Calories

46 Calories • 2 gm Fat • 1 gm Protein •
6 gm Carbohydrate • 116 mg Sodium • 1 mg Calcium •
0 gm Fiber

DIABETIC EXCHANGES: ½ Starch

Quick Raisin Flat Bread

If you've never served piping hot bread for breakfast on a road trip, here's an easy way to change all that. The raisins give this a boost of good-for-you iron, too!   ☻   Serves 8

½ teaspoon ground cinnamon
¼ cup Splenda Granular ☆
1½ cups Bisquick Reduced Fat Baking Mix
¼ cup raisins
½ cup fat-free milk

Preheat oven to 450 degrees. Spray a large baking sheet with butter-flavored cooking spray. In a small bowl, combine cinnamon and 2 tablespoons Splenda. Set aside. In a large bowl, combine baking mix, remaining 2 tablespoons Splenda, and raisins. Add milk. Mix well until mixture forms a soft dough. Spray hands with butter-flavored cooking spray, then pat mixture into an 8-by-8-inch square on prepared baking sheet. Lightly spray top with butter-flavored cooking spray. Evenly sprinkle cinnamon mixture over top. Lightly spray again with butter-flavored spray. Bake for 10 minutes. Cut into 8 servings. Serve hot.

Each serving equals:

HE: 1 Bread • ¼ Fruit • 6 Optional Calories

97 Calories • 1 gm Fat • 2 gm Protein •
20 gm Carbohydrate • 270 mg Sodium •
45 mg Calcium • 1 gm Fiber

DIABETIC EXCHANGES: 1½ Starch/Carbohydrate

Maple Walnut Breakfast Quick Bread

Luscious is the best word I can think of to describe this delectable morning treat. You won't believe how just a dash of walnuts and a smidge of sour cream can work such culinary magic!

◐ Serves 8

> 1½ cups Bisquick Reduced Fat Baking Mix
> ¼ cup Splenda Granular
> ¼ cup (1 ounce) chopped walnuts
> ¼ cup I Can't Believe It's Not Butter! Light Margarine
> ½ cup fat-free milk
> 2 tablespoons Land O Lakes no-fat sour cream
> ½ cup Log Cabin Sugar Free Maple Syrup

Preheat oven to 375 degrees. Spray an 11-by-7-inch biscuit pan with butter-flavored cooking spray. In a large bowl, combine baking mix, Splenda, and walnuts. Add margarine, milk, sour cream, and maple syrup. Mix gently just to combine. Spread batter into prepared biscuit pan. Bake for 14 to 16 minutes. Place pan on a wire rack and let set for at least 5 minutes. Cut into 8 servings.

Each serving equals:

HE: 1 Bread • 1 Fat • ¼ Slider • 10 Optional Calories

146 Calories • 6 gm Fat • 3 gm Protein •
20 gm Carbohydrate • 367 mg Sodium •
51 mg Calcium • 1 gm Fiber

DIABETIC EXCHANGES: 1 Starch • 1 Fat

Apple Pancakes

I chose to use Red Delicious apples in this recipe because they're sturdy and keep well when you're on the road. They're also available in most of the country all year round. But if you find yourself with a Golden Delicious or even a Fuji, give it a try! ● Serves 4

¾ cup Bisquick Reduced Fat Baking Mix
2 teaspoons Splenda Granular
⅓ cup Carnation Nonfat Dry Milk Powder
½ teaspoon apple pie spice
1 egg, beaten, or equivalent in egg substitute
⅔ cup water
½ cup (1 small) cored, unpeeled, and finely diced Red Delicious apple

In a medium bowl, combine baking mix, Splenda, dry milk powder, and apple pie spice. Add egg and water. Mix only until batter is smooth. Fold in apple. Using a ⅓ cup measuring cup as a guide, pour batter onto a hot griddle or skillet sprayed with butter-flavored cooking spray to form 4 pancakes. Cook over medium heat for 1 to 2 minutes on each side or until lightly brown. Serve at once.

HINT: Good served with Log Cabin Sugar Free Maple Syrup or heated unsweetened applesauce. If using either, count accordingly.

Each serving equals:

HE: 1 Bread • ¼ Fat-Free Milk • ¼ Protein • ¼ Fruit • 1 Optional Calorie

131 Calories • 3 gm Fat • 5 gm Protein • 21 gm Carbohydrate • 308 mg Sodium • 94 mg Calcium • 0 gm Fiber

DIABETIC EXCHANGES: 1½ Starch/Carbohydrate

Blueberry Pancakes with Maple Banana Sauce

When we drive along the highway in the summer months, it's always a temptation to stop at roadside stands and buy pints and pints of fresh berries. (Cliff has to remind me sometimes that we'll be passing more stands tomorrow!) This is one of our favorite ways to savor the special flavor of fresh-picked fruit. ○ Serves 6

> 2 tablespoons (½ ounce) chopped pecans
> 1 cup (1 medium) sliced banana
> ½ cup Log Cabin Sugar Free Maple Syrup
> 1½ cups Aunt Jemima Reduced Calorie Pancake Mix
> 2 tablespoons Splenda Granular
> 1 cup water
> ¾ cup fresh blueberries

In a large skillet sprayed with butter-flavored cooking spray, toast pecans for 2 to 3 minutes. Stir in banana slices and maple syrup. Lower heat and simmer while preparing pancakes. In a large bowl, combine pancake mix, Splenda, and water. Gently stir in blueberries. Using a ⅓ cup measuring cup as a guide, drop batter onto a hot griddle or skillet sprayed with butter-flavored cooking spray to form 6 pancakes. Lightly brown pancakes on both sides. For each serving, place a pancake on a plate and spoon about 3 tablespoons banana sauce over top.

Each serving equals:

HE: 1⅓ Bread • ½ Fruit • ⅓ Fat • 15 Optional Calories

---

175 Calories • 3 gm Fat • 7 gm Protein •
30 gm Carbohydrate • 421 mg Sodium •
186 mg Calcium • 5 gm Fiber

DIABETIC EXCHANGES: 1½ Starch • ½ Fruit

Pineapple French Toast

This recipe is almost a microwaveable miracle—it's not only quick and tasty, it's a great way to use up a loaf of bread, and to enjoy a fruity meal that takes only minutes to prepare.

◐ Serves 6 (2 pieces)

> 2 eggs or equivalent in egg substitute
> 1 (8-ounce) can crushed pineapple, packed in fruit juice, undrained
> ¼ cup fat-free milk
> 1 tablespoon Log Cabin Sugar Free Maple Syrup
> 1 tablespoon Splenda Granular
> 1 teaspoon vanilla extract
> 12 slices reduced-calorie day-old white bread

In a blender container, combine eggs, undrained pineapple, milk, maple syrup, Splenda, and vanilla extract. Cover and process on HIGH for 10 seconds or until mixture is smooth. Pour mixture into a shallow dish. Dip bread into egg mixture, coating both sides. Place coated bread slices on a hot griddle or large skillet sprayed with butter-flavored cooking spray. Cook for 3 to 4 minutes on each side or until golden brown.

HINT: Good served with Log Cabin Sugar Free Maple Syrup. If using, count optional calories accordingly.

Each serving equals:

HE: 1 Bread • ½ Protein • ½ Fruit •
6 Optional Calories

---

147 Calories • 3 gm Fat • 8 gm Protein •
22 gm Carbohydrate • 260 mg Sodium •
62 mg Calcium • 1 gm Fiber

DIABETIC EXCHANGES: 1 Starch • ½ Meat • ½ Fruit

Sour Cream French Toast

This might just be the richest, creamiest, most scrumptious French toast you've ever tasted! Yet it's so speedy and easy, you can fix it on a morning when you've got almost no time to eat before you hit the road again. ☻ Serves 2 (2 slices)

> 1 egg, beaten, or equivalent in egg substitute
> 2 tablespoons fat-free milk
> 2 tablespoons Land O Lakes no-fat sour cream
> 2 tablespoons Splenda Granular
> 1 teaspoon ground cinnamon
> 4 slices reduced-calorie white bread

In a shallow bowl, combine egg, milk, and sour cream. Stir in Splenda and cinnamon. Dip bread into egg mixture, coating both sides. Place bread slices on a hot griddle or large skillet sprayed with butter-flavored cooking spray. Cook for 3 to 4 minutes on each side or until golden brown.

HINT: Good served with Log Cabin Sugar Free Maple Syrup or heated unsweetened applesauce. If using either, count accordingly.

Each serving equals:

> HE: 1 Bread • ½ Protein • ¼ Slider •
> 7 Optional Calories
>
> ---
>
> 151 Calories • 3 gm Fat • 9 gm Protein •
> 22 gm Carbohydrate • 290 mg Sodium •
> 96 mg Calcium • 6 gm Fiber
>
> ---
>
> DIABETIC EXCHANGES: 1½ Starch/Carbohydrate •
> ½ Meat

Denver Brunch Bake

Blending all the beloved flavors of a traditional Denver omelette, this party-in-a-pan puffs up beautifully and can turn an ordinary breakfast into an occasion. ❍ Serves 8

2 eggs or equivalent in egg substitute
1/4 cup fat-free milk
2 tablespoons Land O Lakes no-fat sour cream
1 1/2 cups Bisquick Reduced Fat Baking Mix
1 1/2 cups (9 ounces) diced Dubuque 97% fat-free ham or any extra-lean ham
3/4 cup (3 ounces) shredded Kraft reduced-fat Cheddar cheese
1/2 cup chopped onion
1/2 cup chopped green bell pepper

Preheat oven to 350 degrees. Spray a 9-by-9-inch cake pan with butter-flavored cooking spray. In a medium bowl, beat eggs with a fork. Stir in milk and sour cream. Add baking mix, ham, Cheddar cheese, onion, and green pepper. Mix well to combine. Spread mixture evenly into prepared cake pan. Bake for 25 to 30 minutes. Place cake pan on a wire rack and let set for 5 minutes. Cut into 8 servings.

Each serving equals:

HE: 1 1/2 Protein • 1 Bread • 1/4 Vegetable •
6 Optional Calories

169 Calories • 5 gm Fat • 12 gm Protein •
19 gm Carbohydrate • 606 mg Sodium •
116 mg Calcium • 1 gm Fiber

DIABETIC EXCHANGES: 1 1/2 Meat • 1 Starch/Carbohydrate

"Sausage" and Egg Muffins

What I like about muffins is that you can stir just about any combo of ingredients you have on hand into an easy muffin batter. These also freeze and reheat beautifully, so if it's just the two of you, you've got some extra meals ready-made! ☻ Serves 6 (2 each)

> 8 ounces extra-lean ground sirloin beef or turkey breast
> 1/2 teaspoon poultry seasoning
> 1/4 teaspoon ground sage
> 1/4 teaspoon garlic powder
> 3/4 cup (3 ounces) shredded Kraft reduced-fat Cheddar cheese
> 8 eggs or equivalent in egg substitute
> 1/3 cup fat-free milk
> 1 teaspoon dried parsley flakes
> 1/8 teaspoon black pepper

Preheat oven to 375 degrees. Spray a 12-hole muffin pan with butter-flavored cooking spray or line with paper liners. In a large skillet sprayed with butter-flavored cooking spray, brown meat. Stir in poultry seasoning, sage, and garlic powder. Evenly spoon mixture into prepared muffin wells. Sprinkle 1 tablespoon Cheddar cheese over top of each. In a large bowl, beat eggs, milk, parsley flakes, and black pepper using a wire whisk. Pour about 1/4 cup of egg mixture into each muffin cup. Bake for 25 minutes or until a toothpick inserted in center comes out clean. Place muffin pan on a wire rack and let set for 5 minutes. Remove muffins from pan and serve warm.

Each serving equals:

HE: 3 Protein • 5 Optional Calories

178 Calories • 10 gm Fat • 20 gm Protein •
2 gm Carbohydrate • 232 mg Sodium •
145 mg Calcium • 0 gm Fiber

DIABETIC EXCHANGES: 3 Meat

Morning Mix Up

This festive combination is as tummy-filling and taste bud–pleasing as they come! Every bite is just wonderful, with potatoes, cheese, ham, eggs, and onions holding hands and cheering.

◐ Serves 6

> 3 cups (10 ounces) shredded loose-packed frozen potatoes
> ¾ cup finely chopped onion
> 1 full cup (6 ounces) diced Dubuque 97% fat-free ham or any extra-lean ham
> 6 eggs or equivalent in egg substitute
> 1 teaspoon dried parsley flakes
> 1 teaspoon lemon pepper
> ¼ cup + 2 tablespoons (1½ ounces) shredded Kraft reduced-fat Cheddar cheese

In a large skillet sprayed with butter-flavored cooking spray, sauté potatoes, onion, and ham for 10 minutes or until potatoes are tender. In a medium bowl, combine eggs, parsley flakes, and lemon pepper. Pour egg mixture over potato mixture. Continue cooking for 5 minutes or until eggs are set, stirring occasionally. For each serving, spoon full ¾ cup mixture on a plate and sprinkle 1 tablespoon Cheddar cheese over top.

HINT: Mr. Dell's frozen shredded potatoes are a good choice or raw shredded potatoes, rinsed and patted dry, may be used in place of frozen potatoes.

Each serving equals:

HE: 2 Protein • ⅓ Bread • ¼ Vegetable

163 Calories • 7 gm Fat • 14 gm Protein •
11 gm Carbohydrate • 346 mg Sodium •
80 mg Calcium • 1 gm Fiber

DIABETIC EXCHANGES: 2 Meat • ½ Starch

Breakfast Hash

Some days you really long for a hearty breakfast dish, something so full of satisfaction that you're fueled for a busy day ahead. The day I tried this recipe on Cliff, he drove for miles and miles without getting hunger pangs! ☻ Serves 4 (1 cup)

> 8 ounces extra-lean ground sirloin beef or turkey breast
> ½ teaspoon poultry seasoning
> ¼ teaspoon ground sage
> ¼ teaspoon garlic powder
> ¼ cup chopped green bell pepper
> ¼ cup chopped onion
> 2 full cups (12 ounces) diced cooked potatoes
> 3 eggs or equivalent in egg substitute
> 2 tablespoons fat-free milk

In a large skillet sprayed with butter-flavored cooking spray, brown meat, poultry seasoning, sage, garlic powder, green pepper, and onion. Stir in potatoes. Continue cooking for 5 minutes, stirring often. In a medium bowl, combine eggs and milk, using a wire whisk, until blended. Add egg mixture to sausage mixture. Mix well to combine. Continue cooking until eggs are set, stirring occasionally.

Each serving equals:

HE: 2¼ Protein • 1 Bread • ¼ Vegetable • 3 Optional Calories

197 Calories • 9 gm Fat • 16 gm Protein • 13 gm Carbohydrate • 109 mg Sodium • 36 mg Calcium • 1 gm Fiber

DIABETIC EXCHANGES: 2 Meat • 1 Starch

Baked Spanish Potato Omelet

This dish was inspired in part by some leftover potatoes sitting in my fridge. That, and a jar with just a few olives left in it! If you never thought of using potatoes in an egg dish, I hope you'll give this piquant combo a chance some chilly morn.   ☻   Serves 4

> 1½ cups (8 ounces) diced cooked potatoes
> ½ cup chopped green bell pepper
> ½ cup chopped onion
> 6 eggs or equivalent in egg substitute
> 1 (2-ounce) jar chopped pimiento, undrained
> ¼ cup (1 ounce) sliced ripe olives
> ⅛ teaspoon black pepper

Preheat oven to 350 degrees. Spray an 8-by-8-inch baking dish with olive oil–flavored cooking spray. In a large skillet sprayed with olive oil–flavored cooking spray, sauté potatoes, green pepper, and onion for 10 minutes, stirring occasionally. Spoon potato mixture into prepared baking dish. In a medium bowl, combine eggs, undrained pimiento, olives, and black pepper. Pour egg mixture evenly over potato mixture. Bake for 25 to 30 minutes. Place baking dish on a wire rack and let set for 5 minutes. Divide into 4 servings.

Each serving equals:

HE: 1½ Protein • ½ Bread • ½ Vegetable • ¼ Fat

---

164 Calories • 8 gm Fat • 11 gm Protein •
12 gm Carbohydrate • 173 mg Sodium •
54 mg Calcium • 2 gm Fiber

DIABETIC EXCHANGES: 1½ Meat • ½ Starch • ½ Fat

Creamed "Sausage" over English Muffins

If you believed that eating healthy meant giving up the pleasure of sausage in any way, shape, or form, I'm so happy to share this recipe with you! You may not think it's possible to deliver this favorite flavor without the real thing, but the proof is in the tasting.

♥ Serves 4

> 8 ounces extra-lean ground sirloin beef or turkey breast
> 1 (10¾-ounce) can Healthy Request Cream of Mushroom Soup
> ⅓ cup fat-free milk
> 1 (2.5-ounce) can sliced mushrooms, drained
> ½ teaspoon poultry seasoning
> ¼ teaspoon ground sage
> ¼ teaspoon garlic powder
> 1 teaspoon dried onion flakes
> 2 English muffins, split and toasted

In a large skillet sprayed with butter-flavored cooking spray, brown meat. Stir in mushroom soup, milk, mushrooms, poultry seasoning, sage, garlic powder, and onion flakes. Continue cooking until mixture is heated through, stirring often. For each serving, place 1 muffin half on a plate and spoon about ½ cup meat mixture over top.

Each serving equals:

HE: 1½ Protein • 1 Bread • ¼ Vegetable • ½ Slider • 1 Optional Calorie

189 Calories • 5 gm Fat • 15 gm Protein • 21 gm Carbohydrate • 526 mg Sodium • 129 mg Calcium • 1 gm Fiber

DIABETIC EXCHANGES: 1½ Meat • 1½ Starch/Carbohydrate

Ham Scrambled Eggs Benedict

Traditional eggs Benedict calls for Canadian bacon and poached eggs, but the first can be harder to come by when you're traveling, and the second isn't easy to prepare in a moving vehicle! I think this is a wonderful alternative to that more famous version.   ☻   Serves 4

1 (5-ounce) can Hormel lean ham, packed in water, drained and flaked
4 eggs, beaten, or equivalent in egg substitute
¼ cup Land O Lakes no-fat sour cream
¼ cup Kraft fat-free mayonnaise
½ teaspoon Dijon mustard
1 teaspoon lemon juice
1 teaspoon dried parsley flakes
2 English muffins, split and toasted

In a large skillet sprayed with butter-flavored cooking spray, sauté ham for 2 to 3 minutes. Stir in eggs. Continue cooking until eggs are set, stirring often. Meanwhile, in a small saucepan, combine sour cream, mayonnaise, mustard, lemon juice, and parsley flakes. Cook over low heat until scrambled eggs are set, stirring often. For each serving, place a muffin half on a plate, spoon about ½ cup egg mixture over muffin, and top with about 2 tablespoons sauce mixture.

Each serving equals:

HE: 2½ Protein • 1 Bread • ¼ Slider •
5 Optional Calories

---

219 Calories • 8 gm Fat • 15 gm Protein •
19 gm Carbohydrate • 813 mg Sodium •
94 mg Calcium • 1 gm Fiber

DIABETIC EXCHANGES: 2 Meat • 1 Starch

Bacon Rarebit Sauce over Toast

I love "cooking" with prepared bacon bits. I never have to worry about cleaning up pans filled with bacon grease, I get plenty of hearty flavor with fewer calories and less fat, and I've always got bacon in the house. ☻ Serves 6

> 1 (10¾-ounce) can Healthy Request Tomato Soup
> ½ cup nonalcoholic beer or fat-free milk
> ½ cup Hormel Bacon Bits
> 1 teaspoon dried parsley flakes
> ⅛ teaspoon black pepper
> ¾ cup (3 ounces) shredded Kraft reduced-fat Cheddar cheese
> 12 slices reduced-calorie white bread, toasted

In a medium saucepan, combine tomato soup and milk. Stir in bacon bits, parsley flakes, and black pepper. Add Cheddar cheese. Mix well to combine. Cook over medium-low heat for 5 minutes or until mixture is heated through and cheese melts, stirring often. For each serving, place 2 slices of toast on a plate and spoon about ⅓ cup sauce mixture over top.

Each serving equals:

> HE: 1 Bread • ⅔ Protein • ¾ Slider •
> 1 Optional Calorie
>
> ---
>
> 210 Calories • 6 gm Fat • 13 gm Protein •
> 26 gm Carbohydrate • 801 mg Sodium •
> 131 mg Calcium • 1 gm Fiber
>
> ---
>
> DIABETIC EXCHANGES: 1½ Starch/Carbohydrate •
> 1 Meat

Louisiana Eggs Creole

Not everyone is ready for spicy food in the morning, but Cliff always is! This is spicy-flavorful, not spicy-hot, a dish you can serve to any member of the family, and a breakfast entree that will get any day off to a good start.　　❍　　Serves 4

> 8 ounces extra-lean ground sirloin beef or turkey breast
> ½ teaspoon poultry seasoning
> ¼ teaspoon ground sage
> ¼ teaspoon garlic powder
> 1 (8-ounce) can Hunt's Tomato Sauce
> 1 (8-ounce) can stewed tomatoes, finely chopped and undrained
> 6 eggs or equivalent in egg substitute
> ¼ cup fat-free milk
> 1 teaspoon Cajun seasoning
> 8 slices reduced-calorie white bread, toasted

In a large skillet sprayed with butter-flavored cooking spray, brown meat, poultry seasoning, sage, and garlic powder. Add tomato sauce and undrained stewed tomatoes. Mix well to combine. Lower heat and simmer while preparing eggs. In a medium bowl, combine eggs, milk, and Cajun seasoning. Mix well with a fork until blended. Pour egg mixture into a large skillet sprayed with butter-flavored cooking spray. Cook until eggs are set, stirring occasionally. For each serving, place 2 slices toast on a plate, arrange ½ cup scrambled eggs over toast, and spoon about ½ cup meat sauce over top. Serve at once.

Each serving equals:

HE: 3 Protein • 1½ Vegetable • 1 Bread •
6 Optional Calories

298 Calories • 10 gm Fat • 26 gm Protein •
26 gm Carbohydrate • 851 mg Sodium •
119 mg Calcium • 2 gm Fiber

DIABETIC EXCHANGES: 3 Meat • 1½ Vegetable •
1 Starch

Mushroom Scrambled Eggs

Here's a sinfully rich way to serve up scrambled eggs, and once you've stocked your pantry with items like the canned soup and jars of mushrooms, you can whip this recipe up at a moment's notice.

♥ Serves 4 (¾ cup)

> 1 (10¾-ounce) can Healthy Request Cream of Mushroom Soup
> 8 eggs, slightly beaten, or equivalent in egg substitute
> ⅛ teaspoon lemon pepper
> 1 (2.5-ounce) jar sliced mushrooms, drained

In a large bowl, combine mushroom soup, eggs, and lemon pepper. Stir in mushrooms. Pour egg mixture into a large skillet sprayed with butter-flavored cooking spray. Cook over low heat until eggs are set, stirring occasionally.

Each serving equals:

HE: 2 Protein • ¼ Vegetable • ½ Slider •
1 Optional Calorie

---

182 Calories • 10 gm Fat • 14 gm Protein •
9 gm Carbohydrate • 503 mg Sodium •
112 mg Calcium • 0 gm Fiber

DIABETIC EXCHANGES: 2 Meat • ½ Starch/Carbohydrate

Spanish Eggs

You might just think you were listening to a little flamenco music on your CD player when you first taste this savory breakfast dish. (Don't be surprised if at least one family member kicks up his or her heels!)

◑ Serves 2

½ cup diced onion
½ cup diced green bell pepper
½ cup diced celery
1 (8-ounce) can Hunt's Tomato Sauce
¼ teaspoon lemon pepper
3 eggs, beaten, or equivalent in egg substitute
1 tablespoon fat-free milk
1 teaspoon dried parsley flakes

In a medium saucepan sprayed with butter-flavored cooking spray, sauté onion, green pepper, and celery for 6 to 8 minutes or until vegetables are just tender. Add tomato sauce and lemon pepper. Mix well to combine. Lower heat and simmer while preparing eggs. In a medium bowl, combine eggs, milk, and parsley flakes. Pour mixture into a medium skillet sprayed with butter-flavored cooking spray. Cook over medium heat until eggs are set, stirring occasionally. For each serving, place ½ cup egg mixture on plate and spoon ½ cup warm sauce over top.

Each serving equals:

HE: 3½ Vegetable • 1½ Protein • 3 Optional Calories

175 Calories • 7 gm Fat • 12 gm Protein •
16 gm Carbohydrate • 868 mg Sodium •
89 mg Calcium • 3 gm Fiber

DIABETIC EXCHANGES: 3 Vegetable • 1½ Meat

Italian Egg Foo Yung

When the zucchini harvest is under way, I like to stir this healthy veggie into all kinds of dishes, including this unusual take on a familiar egg dish. It's cooked and on the table before you can say "Presto!"
● Serves 4 (¾ cup)

> 2 cups chopped unpeeled zucchini
> ½ cup chopped onion
> 4 eggs or equivalent in egg substitute
> 2 tablespoons Kraft Fat Free Italian Dressing
> ¼ cup Hormel Bacon Bits
> ¼ cup (¾ ounce) Kraft Reduced Fat Parmesan Style Grated
>   Topping

In a large skillet sprayed with olive oil–flavored cooking spray, sauté zucchini and onion for 5 minutes. In a large bowl, combine eggs and Italian dressing. Stir in bacon bits and Parmesan cheese. Add egg mixture to zucchini mixture. Mix well to combine. Lower heat and continue cooking until eggs are set, stirring occasionally.

Each serving equals:

HE: 1¼ Protein • 1¼ Vegetable • ¼ Slider •
9 Optional Calories

---

148 Calories • 8 gm Fat • 11 gm Protein •
8 gm Carbohydrate • 507 mg Sodium •
72 mg Calcium • 1 gm Fiber

DIABETIC EXCHANGES: 2 Meat • 1 Vegetable

Pronto Soups
and Sandwiches

No matter how many miles we're determined to cover on a given travel day, we still have to eat, and often the perfect midday break is for soup and sandwiches in the nearest truckstop parking lot. Depending on the region of the country we're driving through or the availability of certain fresh ingredients, I can stir up a pot of cozy goodness that warms my truck-drivin' man and me to the core. Whenever I sit down to an egg salad sandwich and a mug of homemade soup, I remember long afternoons sitting in my grandma's kitchen, perched on a stool beside the stove. Back then, I stirred the soup with a big wooden spoon and thought about the days to come, when I'd be making soups like this for my own family.

There are an infinite number of delicious combinations in this collection of recipes, so why not start a list of your favorite partners-in-pleasure today? Just think about savoring a steaming bowl of **Easy Seafood Chowder**, coupled with tangy **Thai Tuna Sandwiches**, or maybe you'd rather dig your spoon into a mug of **Jamboree Chili** alongside **Pita Heroes.** You might choose to feast on **Country Calico Stew** while burning up the miles through America's heartland, or after stopping to buy the freshest possible eggs from a roadside stand in dairy country, serve your family my **Eggcellent Egg Salad Sandwiches.** With all these delectable choices up for grabs, your only problem will be deciding which of these tasty treats to fix!

Pronto Soups and Sandwiches

Cheesy Tomato Soup

You get a delicious double-whammy of calcium in this super soup. In fact, with the cheese, you get three—count 'em—three sources of the mineral that helps all of us keep our bones strong.

● Serves 4 (1 cup)

> 1 (12-fluid-ounce) can Carnation Evaporated Fat Free Milk
> 3 tablespoons all-purpose flour
> 3/4 cup (3 ounces) shredded Kraft reduced-fat Cheddar cheese
> 1 cup fat-free milk
> 1 (10 3/4-ounce) can Healthy Request Tomato Soup
> 1/2 teaspoon dried basil

In a covered jar, combine evaporated milk and flour. Shake well to blend. Pour mixture into medium saucepan sprayed with butter-flavored cooking spray. Add Cheddar cheese. Mix well to combine. Cook over medium heat until mixture thickens and cheese melts, stirring constantly. Add milk, tomato soup, and basil. Mix well to combine. Lower heat and simmer for 6 to 8 minutes or until mixture is heated through, stirring constantly.

Each serving equals:

> HE: 1 Fat-Free Milk • 1 Protein • 1/4 Bread •
> 1/2 Slider • 5 Optional Calories
>
> ---
>
> 212 Calories • 4 gm Fat • 16 gm Protein •
> 28 gm Carbohydrate • 550 mg Sodium •
> 506 mg Calcium • 1 gm Fiber
>
> ---
>
> DIABETIC EXCHANGES: 1 Fat-Free Milk • 1 Meat •
> 1 Starch/Carbohydrate

San Antonio Vegetable Soup

As we drove across Texas not long ago on the way to visit my daughter Becky and her family in San Antonio, I found myself thinking of tangy combos inspired by the big tastes Texans truly love. This tasty soup is a true "pantry pleaser," since its major ingredients come straight from the shelf.   ☻   Serves 4 (1 cup)

1/4 cup chopped onion
1 (14 1/2-ounce) can stewed tomatoes, coarsely chopped and
    undrained
3/4 cup water
1 teaspoon chili seasoning
1 (16-ounce) can pinto beans, rinsed and drained
1 (8-ounce) can whole-kernel corn, rinsed and drained
1/4 cup Land O Lakes no-fat sour cream

In a medium saucepan sprayed with butter-flavored cooking spray, sauté onion for 5 minutes. Stir in undrained stewed tomatoes, water, and chili seasoning. Add pinto beans and corn. Mix well to combine. Lower heat and simmer for 6 to 8 minutes or until heated through, stirring occasionally. When serving, top each bowl with 1 tablespoon sour cream.

Each serving equals:

HE: 1 1/4 Protein • 1 Vegetable • 1/2 Bread •
15 Optional Calories

145 Calories • 1 gm Fat • 6 gm Protein •
28 gm Carbohydrate • 532 mg Sodium •
88 mg Calcium • 5 gm Fiber

DIABETIC EXCHANGES: 1 Meat • 1 Vegetable • 1/2 Starch

Vegetable Chili

Like most Americans in recent years, we've tried to put more healthy vegetable dishes on the menu. This veggie chili is completely satisfying without a bit of meat. ☻ Serves 4 (1 cup)

1 (10¾-ounce) can Healthy Request Tomato Soup
1 cup water
1½ teaspoons chili seasoning
1 cup chopped unpeeled zucchini
½ cup shredded carrots
½ cup chopped onion
1 (16-ounce) can red kidney beans, rinsed and drained

In a large saucepan, combine tomato soup, water, and chili seasoning. Add zucchini, carrots, onion, and kidney beans. Mix well to combine. Bring mixture to a boil. Lower heat, cover, and simmer for 30 minutes or until vegetables are tender, stirring occasionally.

Each serving equals:

HE: 1¼ Protein • 1 Vegetable • ½ Slider •
5 Optional Calories

161 Calories • 1 gm Fat • 7 gm Protein •
31 gm Carbohydrate • 298 mg Sodium •
15 mg Calcium • 8 gm Fiber

DIABETIC EXCHANGES: 1 Meat • 1 Vegetable • 1 Starch

Cowboy Soup

You have to drive along dusty rural roads these days to find a true cowboy still driving cattle, but I used my imagination to fix a soul-satisfying dish designed to please the appetites of those hardworking men. ☻ Serves 4 (1 cup)

1 (10¾-ounce) can Healthy Request Tomato Soup
1 (16-ounce) can tomatoes, coarsely chopped and undrained
½ cup water
1 (16-ounce) can pinto beans, rinsed and drained
1 tablespoon Splenda Granular
1 teaspoon dried parsley flakes
2 tablespoons Hormel Bacon Bits

In a large saucepan, combine tomato soup, undrained tomatoes, and water. Add pinto beans, Splenda, and parsley flakes. Mix well to combine. Stir in bacon bits. Cook over medium heat for 10 to 12 minutes or until mixture is heated through, stirring occasionally.

Each serving equals:

HE: 1¼ Protein • 1 Vegetable • ½ Slider • 19 Optional Calories

---

150 Calories • 2 gm Fat • 7 gm Protein • 26 gm Carbohydrate • 622 mg Sodium • 50 mg Calcium • 5 gm Fiber

---

DIABETIC EXCHANGES: 1 Meat • 1 Vegetable • 1 Starch

Tuna Cheese Chowder

There's something so warming about a cheesy soup, I knew I had to try and stir up one that made the most of a handy can of tuna. The surprise here is the tomatoes, but they provide a wonderful flavor and color to a thick and rich chowder.

◐ Serves 4 (1¼ cups)

> ¼ cup finely chopped onion
> 1 (10¾-ounce) can Healthy Request Cream of Mushroom Soup
> 1 cup fat-free milk
> ¾ cup (3 ounces) shredded Kraft reduced-fat Cheddar cheese
> 1 (6-ounce) can white tuna, packed in water, drained and flaked
> 1 teaspoon dried parsley flakes
> 1 (14½-ounce) can stewed tomatoes, coarsely chopped and
>   undrained

In a large saucepan sprayed with butter-flavored cooking spray, sauté onion for 5 minutes. Stir in mushroom soup, milk, and Cheddar cheese. Add tuna and parsley flakes. Mix well to combine. Gradually stir in undrained stewed tomatoes. Lower heat and simmer for 6 to 8 minutes or until cheese melts and mixture is heated through, stirring often.

Each serving equals:

> HE: 1¾ Protein • 1 Vegetable • ¼ Fat-Free Milk •
> ½ Slider • 1 Optional Calorie
>
> ---
>
> 198 Calories • 6 gm Fat • 18 gm Protein •
> 18 gm Carbohydrate • 806 mg Sodium •
> 318 mg Calcium • 1 gm Fiber
>
> ---
>
> DIABETIC EXCHANGES: 2 Meat • 1 Vegetable •
> ½ Starch

Easy Seafood Chowder

You don't have to be on either coast to enjoy the bounty of the ocean. The combination of shrimp and tuna in this creamy chowder may convince you that you'll be at the beach by sunrise.

● Serves 4 (1¼ cups)

> 1 cup chopped onion
> 1½ cups (8 ounces) diced cooked potatoes
> 1 (10¾-ounce) can Healthy Request Cream of Celery Soup
> 1⅓ cups fat-free milk
> ½ teaspoon dried dill weed
> 1 (4.5-ounce drained weight) can medium shrimp, rinsed and
>   drained
> 1 (6-ounce) can white tuna, packed in water, drained and flaked

In a large saucepan sprayed with butter-flavored cooking spray, sauté onion for 5 minutes or until tender. Stir in potatoes, celery soup, milk, and dill weed. Add shrimp and tuna. Mix well to combine. Lower heat and simmer for 10 minutes, stirring occasionally.

Each serving equals:

HE: 2½ Protein • ½ Bread • ½ Vegetable •
⅓ Fat-Free Milk • ½ Slider • 1 Optional Calorie

203 Calories • 3 gm Fat • 23 gm Protein •
21 gm Carbohydrate • 544 mg Sodium •
188 mg Calcium • 1 gm Fiber

DIABETIC EXCHANGES: 2½ Meat • 1 Starch •
½ Vegetable

Country Chicken Chowder

Here's a soup that celebrates all the goodness of America in one big bowl, with the bounty of the heartland sharing the stage!

● Serves 4 (1½ cups)

> 1 cup finely chopped celery
> ½ cup chopped onion
> 1 (10¾-ounce) can Healthy Request Cream of Chicken Soup
> 1 (12-fluid-ounce) can Carnation Evaporated Fat Free Milk
> ¾ cup water
> 1 teaspoon dried parsley flakes
> 1 (8-ounce) can whole-kernel corn, rinsed and drained
> 1½ cups (8 ounces) diced cooked potatoes
> 1 cup (5 ounces) diced cooked chicken breast
> ¼ cup Hormel Bacon Bits

In a large saucepan sprayed with butter-flavored cooking spray, sauté celery and onion for 6 to 8 minutes. Stir in chicken soup, evaporated milk, water, and parsley flakes. Add corn, potatoes, chicken, and bacon bits. Mix well to combine. Lower heat and simmer for 5 minutes or until mixture is heated through, stirring occasionally.

HINT: If you don't have leftovers, purchase a chunk of cooked chicken breast from your local deli or use a 5-ounce can of chicken breast, packed in water.

Each serving equals:

HE: 1¼ Protein • 1 Bread • ¾ Fat-Free Milk • ¾ Vegetable • ¾ Slider • 10 Optional Calories

288 Calories • 4 gm Fat • 24 gm Protein • 39 gm Carbohydrate • 774 mg Sodium • 265 mg Calcium • 3 gm Fiber

DIABETIC EXCHANGES: 2 Meat • 1½ Starch • 1 Fat-Free Milk • ½ Vegetable

Oriental Chicken Soup

You can usually find great soups at just about any Chinese restaurant, but if you're on a stretch of road that hasn't got a single one, you can still enjoy the flavors you crave, with this chicken charmer. The rice plumps beautifully in the broth.   ● Serves 4 (1½ cups)

> 1 (16-ounce) can Healthy Request Chicken Broth
> 1 cup water
> 3 cups frozen stir-fry vegetables
> 1 (10¾-ounce) can Healthy Request Cream of Chicken Soup
> 1 (5-ounce) can Hormel 97% Fat Free Breast of Chicken, packed in
>   water, drained and flaked
> 1 (2.5-ounce) jar sliced mushrooms, drained
> 2 teaspoons Oriental seasoning
> ⅔ cup (2 ounces) uncooked Minute Rice

In a large saucepan, combine chicken broth, water, and frozen vegetables. Bring mixture to a boil. Stir in chicken soup, chicken, mushrooms, and Oriental seasoning. Lower heat and simmer for 5 minutes. Add uncooked rice. Mix well to combine. Cover and continue simmering for 10 minutes or until rice and vegetables are tender, stirring occasionally.

Each serving equals:

> HE: 1¾ Vegetable • 1¼ Protein • ½ Bread •
> ½ Slider • 13 Optional Calories
>
> ---
>
> 208 Calories • 4 gm Fat • 15 gm Protein •
> 28 gm Carbohydrate • 711 mg Sodium •
> 84 mg Calcium • 4 gm Fiber
>
> ---
>
> DIABETIC EXCHANGES: 1½ Vegetable • 1 Meat •
> 1 Starch/Carbohydrate

Corn and Chicken Noodle Soup

There's probably not a more beloved pair in soups than a chicken and noodles duet. But if two makes for nice company, why not invite a crowd into your cookpot, with the addition of creamy corn that makes beautiful music with the rest!

 ☻   Serves 4 (1¼ cups)

> 1 (5-ounce) can Hormel 97% Fat Free Breast of Chicken, packed in
>   water, drained and flaked
> 1 (16-ounce) can Healthy Request Chicken Broth
> 1 cup water
> ¾ cup chopped celery
> ¼ cup chopped onion
> 1 (8-ounce) can cream-style corn
> Scant 1 cup (1½ ounces) uncooked noodles
> 2 teaspoons dried parsley flakes
> ⅛ teaspoon black pepper

In a medium saucepan, combine chicken, chicken broth, water, celery, and onion. Bring mixture to a boil. Lower heat, cover, and simmer for 15 to 20 minutes or until vegetables are tender. Stir in corn, uncooked noodles, parsley flakes, and black pepper. Cover and continue simmering for 15 minutes or until noodles are tender, stirring occasionally.

Each serving equals:

HE: 1¼ Protein • 1 Bread • ½ Vegetable •
16 Optional Calories

---

176 Calories • 4 gm Fat • 12 gm Protein •
23 gm Carbohydrate • 624 mg Sodium •
24 mg Calcium • 2 gm Fiber

DIABETIC EXCHANGES: 1½ Starch • 1 Meat

Smoked-Turkey Bean Soup

Soup is one of our favorite lunch choices when we're traveling on a book tour. Soup's filling, of course, and it's easy to reheat leftovers in the microwave. But the best reason for choosing this hale and hearty dish is the flavor it delivers in every mouthful.

☻ Serves 4 (1¼ cups)

> 1 (16-ounce) can Healthy Request Chicken Broth
> ½ cup chopped onion
> 1 cup shredded carrots
> ½ cup diced celery
> 1 (10¾-ounce) can Healthy Request Cream of Chicken Soup
> 1 (16-ounce) can great northern beans, rinsed and drained
> 1 (6-ounce) package Healthy Choice 97% fat-free smoked turkey breast, diced
> 1 teaspoon dried parsley flakes

In a large saucepan, combine chicken broth, onion, carrots, and celery. Bring mixture to a boil. Stir in chicken soup, great northern beans, turkey, and parsley flakes. Lower heat, cover, and simmer for 15 minutes or until vegetables are tender, stirring occasionally.

Each serving equals:

> HE: 2¼ Protein • 1 Vegetable • ½ Slider •
> 13 Optional Calories
>
> ---
>
> 185 Calories • 1 gm Fat • 15 gm Protein •
> 29 gm Carbohydrate • 879 mg Sodium •
> 55 mg Calcium • 5 gm Fiber
>
> ---
>
> DIABETIC EXCHANGES: 2 Meat • 1 Vegetable • 1 Starch

Country Ham–Corn Chowder

This dish practically stands up and sings the Iowa state song, with all that corn in every spoonful! It's an old-fashioned recipe that's sure to appeal to all those long-distance drivers who cross the Midwest every day of the year.　 ☻　 Serves 6 (1 cup)

3 cups (18 ounces) diced
　Dubuque 97% fat-free
　ham or any extra-lean
　ham
2 cups (10 ounces) diced raw
　potatoes
1 cup finely chopped celery
½ cup chopped onion
1 (16-ounce) can Healthy
　Request Chicken Broth

1 (8-ounce) can cream-style
　corn
1 (8-ounce) can whole-kernel
　corn, rinsed and drained
2 teaspoons dried parsley flakes
⅛ teaspoon black pepper
1 cup Carnation Nonfat Dry
　Milk Powder
1 cup water

In a large saucepan, combine ham, potatoes, celery, onion, and chicken broth. Bring mixture to a boil. Stir in cream-style corn, whole-kernel corn, parsley flakes, and black pepper. Lower heat, cover, and simmer for 15 minutes or until potatoes are tender, stirring occasionally. In a small bowl, combine dry milk powder and water. Add milk mixture to soup mixture. Mix well to combine. Continue simmering for 5 to 6 minutes or until mixture is heated through, stirring occasionally.

Each serving equals:

HE: 2 Protein • 1 Bread • ½ Fat-Free Milk •
½ Vegetable • 6 Optional Calories

231 Calories • 3 gm Fat • 21 gm Protein •
30 gm Carbohydrate • 809 mg Sodium •
162 mg Calcium • 2 gm Fiber

DIABETIC EXCHANGES: 2 Meat • 1 Starch •
½ Fat Free Milk • ½ Vegetable

Cheesy Potato Ham Soup

Isn't it great to know we don't have to give up cheese soup when we decide to eat healthy? You won't be able to tell the difference between the "light" version and the original, but you'll know you're eating something really good—and good for you!

● Serves 4 (1½ cups)

> 3 cups (15 ounces) diced raw potatoes
> 1 cup shredded carrots
> ½ cup finely diced onion
> 1 cup water
> 1 (10¾-ounce) can Healthy Request Cream of Celery Soup
> 1 cup fat-free milk
> ¾ cup (3 ounces) cubed Velveeta Light processed cheese
> 1 full cup (6 ounces) diced Dubuque 97% fat-free ham or any
>   extra-lean ham

In an 8-cup microwavable bowl, combine potatoes, carrots, onion, and water. Cover and microwave on HIGH (100% power) for 4 to 5 minutes or until potatoes are tender, stirring occasionally. Partially mash vegetables, using a potato masher or fork. Stir in celery soup and milk. Add Velveeta cheese and ham. Mix well to combine. Re-cover and microwave on HIGH for 4 minutes or until mixture is hot and cheese is melted, stirring after 2 minutes.

Each serving equals:

HE: 2 Protein • ¾ Bread • ¾ Vegetable •
¼ Fat-Free Milk • ½ Slider • 1 Optional Calorie

---

245 Calories • 5 gm Fat • 16 gm Protein •
34 gm Carbohydrate • 914 mg Sodium •
278 mg Calcium • 3 gm Fiber

DIABETIC EXCHANGES: 2 Meat • 1½ Starch • 1 Vegetable

Jamboree Chili

When all the scouts get together to celebrate, it's called a jamboree.
When all the flavors in this dish set up camp side-by-side, it's called
a dish to delight! ☻ Serves 4 (1 cup)

8 ounces extra-lean ground sirloin beef or turkey breast
½ cup chopped onion
1 (16-ounce) can red kidney beans, rinsed and drained
1 (15-ounce) can Hunt's Tomato Sauce
1 cup chunky salsa (mild, medium, or hot)
1 teaspoon chili seasoning

In a medium saucepan sprayed with olive oil–flavored cooking
spray, brown meat and onion. Add kidney beans, tomato sauce, salsa,
and chili seasoning. Mix well to combine. Lower heat and simmer for
10 minutes, stirring occasionally.

Each serving equals:

HE: 2½ Vegetable • 1½ Protein • 1¼ Bread

193 Calories • 5 gm Fat • 15 gm Protein •
22 gm Carbohydrate • 924 mg Sodium •
116 mg Calcium • 6 gm Fiber

DIABETIC EXCHANGES: 2 Meat • 2 Vegetable • ½ Starch

Beefy Mushroom–White Bean Soup

Does it shock you to find Bisquick in a beefy soup blend? It's a smart cook's secret for thickening a hearty soup without making it too heavy. This is a real man-pleaser, healthy *and* filling.

⊙   Serves 4 (1¼ cups)

> 8 ounces extra-lean ground sirloin beef or turkey breast
> 2 cups chopped fresh mushrooms
> 1 (16-ounce) can great northern beans, rinsed and drained
> 1 (14½-ounce) can Swanson Beef Broth
> 3 tablespoons Bisquick Reduced Fat Baking Mix
> 1 teaspoon dried parsley flakes
> 1 cup water

In a large saucepan sprayed with butter-flavored cooking spray, brown meat and mushrooms. Stir in great northern beans. In a covered jar, combine beef broth, baking mix, and parsley flakes. Shake well to blend. Stir broth mixture and water into saucepan with meat mixture. Continue cooking for 5 to 7 minutes or until mixture thickens, stirring often.

Each serving equals:

> HE: 2¾ Protein • 1 Vegetable • ¼ Bread •
> 8 Optional Calories
>
> ---
>
> 188 Calories • 4 gm Fat • 18 gm Protein •
> 20 gm Carbohydrate • 453 mg Sodium •
> 46 mg Calcium • 4 gm Fiber
>
> ---
>
> DIABETIC EXCHANGES: 2 Meat • 1 Starch • ½ Vegetable

Country Calico Stew

Skillet suppers are great for on-the-road meals because they don't require a lot of time or demand dishwashing that never ends! This dish invites a crowd of flavors into one hot pan, and the result: a sizzler that satisfies everyone at the table. ☉ Serves 4 (1 cup)

> 8 ounces extra-lean ground sirloin beef or turkey breast
> 1 (10¾-ounce) can Healthy Request Tomato Soup
> ¼ cup water
> ½ teaspoon poultry seasoning
> ¼ teaspoon ground sage
> ¼ teaspoon garlic powder
> 1 cup (5 ounces) diced cooked chicken breast
> 1 (8-ounce) can whole-kernel corn, rinsed and drained
> 1½ cups (8 ounces) diced cooked potatoes

In a large skillet sprayed with butter-flavored cooking spray, brown meat. Stir in tomato soup, water, poultry seasoning, sage, and garlic powder. Add chicken, corn, and potatoes. Mix well to combine. Lower heat and simmer for 6 to 8 minutes or until mixture is heated through, stirring occasionally.

HINT: If you don't have leftovers, purchase a chunk of cooked chicken breast from your local deli or use a 5-ounce can of chicken breast, packed in water.

Each serving equals:

HE: 2¾ Protein • 1 Bread • ½ Slider •
5 Optional Calories

---

259 Calories • 7 gm Fat • 24 gm Protein •
25 gm Carbohydrate • 314 mg Sodium •
18 mg Calcium • 2 gm Fiber

DIABETIC EXCHANGES: 3 Meat • 1½ Starch

Summer Tomato-Cheese Sandwiches

I'm so proud of my own tomato harvest, I hate to be on the road during the weeks when my ruby-red treasures are just about ripe. But if we're not home to eat tomatoes from my garden, you can be sure we're eating them everywhere else!   ☻   Serves 4

> ⅓ cup Kraft fat-free mayonnaise
> ½ teaspoon lemon pepper
> 2 tablespoons Hormel Bacon Bits
> 8 slices reduced-calorie sourdough bread, toasted
> 1 cup sliced ripe tomatoes
> ½ cup finely shredded lettuce
> 4 (¾-ounce) slices reduced-fat American cheese

In a small bowl, combine mayonnaise, lemon pepper, and bacon bits. Spread a scant tablespoon of mayonnaise mixture on slices of toast. Top 4 slices each with ¼ cup sliced tomatoes, 2 tablespoons lettuce, 1 slice American cheese, and another slice of toast, mayonnaise side down. Cut each sandwich in half diagonally. Serve at once.

Each serving equals:

HE: 1 Bread • 1 Protein • ¾ Vegetable • ¼ Slider • 6 Optional Calories

176 Calories • 4 gm Fat • 10 gm Protein • 25 gm Carbohydrate • 939 mg Sodium • 162 mg Calcium • 2 gm Fiber

DIABETIC EXCHANGES: 1 Starch • 1 Meat • ½ Vegetable

Sunshine Special Sandwiches

Carrot salads turn up at almost every potluck supper, but why not try mounding this fresh and fruity salad, so rich with vitamin A, on your favorite bun for a change of pace?   ☻   Serves 4

    1 cup shredded carrots
    ¼ cup (1 ounce) chopped walnuts
    ½ cup raisins
    ⅓ cup Kraft fat-free mayonnaise
    1 teaspoon lemon juice
    1 tablespoon Splenda Granular
    4 small hamburger buns

In a medium bowl, combine carrots, walnuts, and raisins. Add mayonnaise, lemon juice, and Splenda. Mix well to combine. For each sandwich, spoon a full ⅓ cup mixture between each hamburger bun. Serve at once or cover and refrigerate until ready to serve.

Each serving equals:

    HE: 1 Bread • 1 Fruit • ½ Fat • ½ Vegetable •
    ¼ Protein • 15 Optional Calories

    _____

    206 Calories • 6 gm Fat • 4 gm Protein •
    34 gm Carbohydrate • 343 mg Sodium •
    26 mg Calcium • 3 gm Fiber

    _____

    DIABETIC EXCHANGES: 1 Starch • 1 Fruit • 1 Fat

Eggcellent Egg Salad Sandwiches

Just as I couldn't resist the pun in this recipe's title, my taste testers couldn't resist the festive blend of bacon and eggs in this special sandwich. Even when you think you know what to expect from an egg salad sandwich, you find you can still be surprised!

❂ Serves 4

>   4 hard-boiled eggs, chopped
>   ¼ cup Kraft fat-free mayonnaise
>   2 teaspoons Dijon mustard
>   1 tablespoon sweet pickle relish
>   2 tablespoons Hormel Bacon Bits
>   1 tablespoon chopped black olives
>   4 lettuce leaves
>   8 slices reduced-calorie white bread

In a medium bowl, combine chopped eggs, mayonnaise, mustard, and pickle relish. Add bacon bits and olives. Mix gently to combine. For each sandwich, arrange a lettuce leaf over a slice of bread, spread ⅓ cup egg mixture over lettuce, and top with another slice of bread. Serve at once or cover and refrigerate until ready to serve.

Each serving equals:

HE: 1 Bread • 1 Protein • ¼ Slider •
6 Optional Calories

---

198 Calories • 6 gm Fat • 13 gm Protein •
23 gm Carbohydrate • 653 mg Sodium •
63 mg Calcium • 5 gm Fiber

DIABETIC EXCHANGES: 1½ Starch/Carbohydrate • 1 Meat

Dilled Egg Salad Sandwiches

There's something so comforting about egg salad sandwiches—maybe because our moms always made them for us for school lunches? This recipe is a perfect example of how to make a good thing just that little bit better. For me, it's the lemon pepper and dill pickle relish that make a favorite sandwich a special event!

◑ Serves 4

> 6 hard-boiled eggs, chopped
> ½ cup finely chopped celery
> ½ cup Kraft fat-free mayonnaise
> 2 tablespoons dill pickle relish
> 1 (2-ounce) jar diced pimiento, drained
> ¼ teaspoon lemon pepper
> 1 cup shredded lettuce
> 8 slices reduced-calorie bread

In a medium bowl, combine eggs and celery. Add mayonnaise, dill pickle relish, pimiento, and lemon pepper. Mix gently to combine. For each sandwich, place ¼ cup lettuce on a slice of bread, spoon ½ cup egg mixture over lettuce, and top with another slice of bread. Serve at once or cover and refrigerate until ready to serve.

Each serving equals:

HE: 1½ Protein • 1 Bread • ½ Vegetable • ¼ Slider

220 Calories • 8 gm Fat • 14 gm Protein •
23 gm Carbohydrate • 606 mg Sodium •
89 mg Calcium • 1 gm Fiber

DIABETIC EXCHANGES: 1½ Meat • 1 Starch •
½ Vegetable

San Antonio Egg Salad Rollups

I love the ease of wrapped sandwiches, and as long as I have a package of refrigerated tortillas, I'm ready to roll! Tangy salsa makes a splendid (if surprising) partner for classic egg salad in this taste-as-big-as-Texas treat.   ☺   Serves 4

4 hard-boiled eggs, finely chopped
½ cup chunky salsa (mild, medium, or hot)
¼ cup Kraft fat-free mayonnaise
1 teaspoon dried parsley flakes
4 (6-inch) flour tortillas

In a medium bowl, combine eggs, salsa, mayonnaise, and parsley flakes. Refrigerate until ready to serve. Just before serving, warm tortillas in microwave or oven and evenly spoon a full ⅓ cup egg mixture into center of each. Roll up. Serve at once or cover and refrigerate until ready to serve.

Each serving equals:

HE: 1 Bread • 1 Protein • ¼ Vegetable •
10 Optional Calories

216 Calories • 8 gm Fat • 10 gm Protein •
26 gm Carbohydrate • 577 mg Sodium •
86 mg Calcium • 2 gm Fiber

DIABETIC EXCHANGES: 1 Starch • 1 Meat

Thai Tuna Sandwiches

One of the delectable surprises of Asian cuisine is a touch of peanut flavor in many dishes. Here, where you might never expect to find it, is a tuna sandwich with a savory difference!   ☻   Serves 4

½ cup Kraft fat-free mayonnaise
2 tablespoons Peter Pan reduced-fat crunchy peanut butter
1 (6-ounce) can white tuna, packed in water, drained and flaked
1 teaspoon dried onion flakes
8 slices reduced-calorie wheat bread
½ cup finely shredded lettuce

In a medium bowl, combine mayonnaise and peanut butter. Stir in tuna and onion flakes. For each sandwich, spread ¼ cup tuna mixture on a slice of bread, sprinkle 2 tablespoons lettuce over filling, and top with another slice of bread.

HINT: Peanut butter spreads best at room temperature.

Each serving equals:

HE: 1¼ Protein • 1 Bread • ½ Fat • ¼ Vegetable • ¼ Slider

267 Calories • 3 gm Fat • 19 gm Protein •
41 gm Carbohydrate • 810 mg Sodium •
57 mg Calcium • 5 gm Fiber

DIABETIC EXCHANGES: 2 Meat • 1½ Starch/Carbohydrate

Chicken Waldorf Sandwich

Waldorf salad is a delicious hotel classic, but I thought it would be fun take it out of the kitchen and onto the road! It's rich and crunchy all at once, a terrific choice for lunch on the run.

❤ Serves 4

> 1 cup (5 ounces) diced cooked chicken breast
> ½ cup chopped celery
> ½ cup (1 small) cored and chopped apple
> ¼ cup (1 ounce) chopped walnuts
> ⅓ cup Kraft fat-free mayonnaise
> 1 teaspoon lemon juice
> 4 lettuce leaves
> 4 small hamburger buns

In a medium bowl, combine chicken, celery, apple, and walnuts. Add mayonnaise and lemon juice. Mix well to combine. For each sandwich, place a lettuce leaf and ½ cup chicken mixture between each hamburger bun. Serve at once or cover and refrigerate until ready to serve.

HINT: If you don't have leftovers, purchase a chunk of cooked chicken breast from your local deli or use a 5-ounce can of chicken breast, packed in water.

Each serving equals:

HE: 1½ Protein • 1 Bread • ½ Fat • ¼ Fruit • ¼ Vegetable • 8 Optional Calories

203 Calories • 7 gm Fat • 14 gm Protein • 21 gm Carbohydrate • 331 mg Sodium • 26 mg Calcium • 2 gm Fiber

DIABETIC EXCHANGES: 1½ Meat • 1½ Starch/Carbohydrate • 1 Fat

BBQ Turkey Sandwiches

These crunchy delights take minutes to prepare, but they deliver the kind of flavor you wouldn't expect from a speedy sandwich. The cabbage adds some delectable color and texture.   ☻   Serves 4

> 1 (6-ounce) package Healthy Choice deli sliced turkey breast,
>   shredded
> 2 teaspoons dried onion flakes
> ½ cup Healthy Choice Barbecue Sauce
> 1 cup shredded cabbage
> 4 small hamburger buns

In a large skillet sprayed with butter-flavored cooking spray, combine turkey, onion flakes, and barbecue sauce. Cook over medium heat for 5 to 6 minutes, stirring often. For each sandwich, place ¼ cup cabbage on bun bottom, spoon ¼ cup meat mixture on top, and cover with bun top. Serve at once.

Each serving equals:

HE: 1 Protein • 1 Bread • ½ Vegetable • ½ Slider • 10 Optional Calories

139 Calories • 2 gm Fat • 9 gm Protein • 21 gm Carbohydrate • 917 mg Sodium • 18 mg Calcium • 2 gm Fiber

DIABETIC EXCHANGES: 1½ Starch/Carbohydrate • 1 Meat • ½ Vegetable

Tom's Ham and Swiss Bagel Sandwich

If I asked my son Tom what he wanted for lunch, I'd get the same answer just about every time: ham and swiss! But once he tasted this beauty on a bagel, he started asking for "ham and swiss with that cucumber stuff!" ☺ Serves 4

> 1 teaspoon dried onion flakes
> 2 tablespoons white distilled vinegar
> 2 teaspoons Splenda Granular
> ½ cup thinly sliced cucumbers
> 4 (¾-ounce) slices Kraft reduced-fat Swiss cheese
> 4 small onion-flavored bagels
> 1 (2.5-ounce) package Carl Buddig 97% fat-free ham
> 2 tablespoons Kraft fat-free mayonnaise

In a small bowl, combine onion flakes, vinegar, Splenda, and cucumbers. Cover and refrigerate for at least 1 hour. Just before serving, place 1 slice cheese on bottom half of each bagel. Evenly divide ham and arrange over cheese slice. Evenly arrange cucumber slices over ham. Spread ½ tablespoon mayonnaise on cut side of bagel top. Arrange top over cucumbers. Serve at once or cover and refrigerate until ready to serve.

Each serving equals:

HE: 2 Bread • 1½ Protein • ¼ Vegetable • 6 Optional Calories

283 Calories • 7 gm Fat • 17 gm Protein • 38 gm Carbohydrate • 748 mg Sodium • 232 mg Calcium • 2 gm Fiber

DIABETIC EXCHANGES: 2 Starch • 1½ Meat

Pita Heroes

You can now find pita bread in grocery stores from the Deep South to the Far West, so finding wonderful ways to fill this Middle Eastern bread has been one of my passions in recent years. This take-along ham and cheese combo is a winner in any season, but especially good with summer-fresh tomatoes.   ☻   Serves 4

> 1 cup finely shredded lettuce
> 1 full cup (6 ounces) diced Dubuque 97% fat-free ham or any
>   extra-lean ham
> ½ cup diced fresh tomatoes
> 2 (¾-ounce) slices Kraft reduced-fat Swiss cheese, shredded
> ½ cup Kraft Free Classic Caesar Dressing
> 2 pita rounds, halved

In a medium bowl, combine lettuce, ham, tomatoes, and Swiss cheese. Add Classic Caesar dressing. Mix gently to combine. Spoon about ⅔ cup filling mixture into each pita half. Serve at once or cover and refrigerate until ready to serve.

HINT: To make opening pita rounds easier, place pita halves on a paper towel and microwave on HIGH 10 seconds. Remove and gently press open.

Each serving equals:

HE: 1½ Protein • 1 Bread • ½ Vegetable • ½ Slider •
10 Optional Calories

212 Calories • 4 gm Fat • 14 gm Protein •
30 gm Carbohydrate • 875 mg Sodium •
128 mg Calcium • 2 gm Fiber

DIABETIC EXCHANGES: 1½ Meat • 1½ Starch •
½ Vegetable

Chili Burgers

My kids just loved this version of chili-on-a-bun, and I bet your loved ones will jump on the bandwagon too! It's a quick and hearty meal for all year round, and perfect with a cup of tomato soup on the side. ☻ Serves 4

8 ounces extra-lean ground sirloin beef or turkey breast
½ cup chopped onion
½ cup chopped green bell pepper
1 (8-ounce) can Hunt's Tomato Sauce
1 (16-ounce) can pinto beans, rinsed and drained
2 teaspoons chili seasoning
1 tablespoon Splenda Granular
1 teaspoon dried parsley flakes
4 small hamburger buns

In a large skillet sprayed with olive oil–flavored cooking spray, brown meat, onion, and green pepper. Stir in tomato sauce and pinto beans. Add chili seasoning, Splenda, and parsley flakes. Mix well to combine. Lower heat and simmer for 5 minutes. For each serving, spoon about ⅔ cup meat mixture between each hamburger bun.

Each serving equals:

HE: 2¾ Protein • 1½ Vegetable • 1 Bread • 1 Optional Calorie

241 Calories • 5 gm Fat • 18 gm Protein • 31 gm Carbohydrate • 657 mg Sodium • 50 mg Calcium • 6 gm Fiber

DIABETIC EXCHANGES: 2 Meat • 1½ Starch • 1½ Vegetable

Pan Burgers

Sure, you could stop for fast-food burgers in Anytown, USA, but if you and your family have a hankering for a more substantial burger taste, here's a homemade version you can sizzle in your skillet—or pop onto the barbecue if you're camped at a national park!

○ Serves 6

16 ounces extra-lean ground sirloin beef or turkey breast
½ cup (1½-ounces) quick oats
1 teaspoon Worcestershire sauce
1 teaspoon prepared yellow mustard
2 tablespoons reduced-sodium ketchup
1 teaspoon dried onion flakes
6 small hamburger buns

In a large bowl, combine meat, oats, Worcestershire sauce, mustard, ketchup, and onion flakes. Using a ⅓ cup measuring cup as a guide, form into 6 patties. Place patties in a large skillet sprayed with butter-flavored cooking spray. Brown for 4 to 6 minutes on each side. For each sandwich, place 1 patty between each hamburger bun.

Each serving equals:

HE: 2 Protein • 1⅓ Bread • 5 Optional Calories

197 Calories • 5 gm Fat • 18 gm Protein •
20 gm Carbohydrate • 223 mg Sodium •
9 mg Calcium • 2 gm Fiber

DIABETIC EXCHANGES: 2 Meat • 1½ Starch

Quick Skillet Burgers

You'll notice I suggest either ground sirloin or ground turkey breast in many of my recipes. If you always choose the beef, why not travel new ground tonight and try some tangy turkey for a change?

○ Serves 6

> 16 ounces extra-lean ground sirloin beef or turkey breast
> ½ cup onion
> ¼ cup chopped green bell pepper
> 1 (10¾-ounce) can Healthy Request Tomato Soup
> 1 teaspoon chili seasoning
> 6 small hamburger buns

In a large skillet sprayed with olive oil–flavored cooking spray, brown meat, onion, and green pepper. Stir in tomato soup and chili seasoning. Lower heat and simmer for 5 minutes, stirring occasionally. For each sandwich, spoon about ½ cup meat mixture between each hamburger bun.

Each serving equals:

HE: 2 Protein • 1 Bread • ¼ Vegetable • ¼ Slider • 10 Optional Calories

---

220 Calories • 8 gm Fat • 16 gm Protein • 21 gm Carbohydrate • 385 mg Sodium • 11 mg Calcium • 2 gm Fiber

---

DIABETIC EXCHANGES: 2 Meat • 1 Starch

Easy Barbecued Sandwiches

There's no time to fire up the grill, but that doesn't mean you have to give up the savory barbecue flavor you love so much. I made Cliff keep taste-testing the sauce for this skillet supper until he pronounced it just about perfect!   ○   Serves 6

16 ounces extra-lean ground sirloin beef or turkey breast
¾ cup finely chopped onion
½ cup reduced-sodium ketchup
⅓ cup sweet pickle relish
6 small hamburger buns

In a large skillet sprayed with butter-flavored cooking spray, brown meat and onion. Add ketchup and pickle relish. Mix well to combine. Lower heat and simmer for 6 to 8 minutes, stirring occasionally. For each sandwich, spoon scant ½ cup meat sauce between each hamburger bun.

Each serving equals:

HE: 2 Protein • 1 Bread • ¼ Vegetable • ¼ Slider • 13 Optional Calories

213 Calories • 5 gm Fat • 17 gm Protein • 25 gm Carbohydrate • 317 mg Sodium • 10 mg Calcium • 2 gm Fiber

DIABETIC EXCHANGES: 2 Meat • 1½ Starch/Carbohydrate

Teriyaki Burgers

With many international dishes, it's the spices that sing with the music of an exotic locale. Just a bit of ginger turns a basic burger into a culinary excursion, a mini-vacation across the Pacific with every scrumptious bite!   ☯   Serves 6

> 16 ounces extra-lean ground sirloin beef or turkey breast
> 6 tablespoons purchased graham cracker crumbs or 6 (2½-inch)
>   graham cracker squares made into crumbs
> ⅛ teaspoon ground ginger
> 1 teaspoon dried parsley flakes
> 2 tablespoons reduced-sodium soy sauce
> 2 tablespoons water

In a large bowl, combine meat, cracker crumbs, ginger, parsley flakes, soy sauce, and water. Mix well to combine. Using a ⅓ cup measuring cup as a guide, form into 6 patties. Place patties in a large skillet sprayed with butter-flavored cooking spray. Brown for 4 to 6 minutes on each side. Serve as is or on hamburger buns.

HINT: A self-seal sandwich bag works great for crushing crackers.

Each serving equals:

HE: 2 Protein • ⅓ Bread

---

233 Calories • 9 gm Fat • 15 gm Protein •
23 gm Carbohydrate • 420 mg Sodium •
1 mg Calcium • 1 gm Fiber

DIABETIC EXCHANGES: 2 Meat • ½ Starch

Quick Side Dishes

In a movie, it's often the players whose names appear far down in the credits who make the most memorable impression, and the same is true when it's time for a potluck celebration with family and friends. Sure, everyone pays attention to the entree, but it's all those tasty side dishes that win their hearts—the coleslaw, the potato salad, the relishes, and the vegetable casseroles that lend so much color and flavor to your table. These are the recipes handed down through the generations, just as my own mother and grandmother entrusted their favorites to me. When I recall picnics by the riverside, I remember what we ate as vividly as who shared our repast!

When you're having dinner at my house or pulling up a lawn chair to my motor home for an impromptu meal, you'll never be handed a plate containing just one or two items! It's my family tradition—and Cliff's expectation—that I'll be serving several different side dishes along with the main event. If it's midsummer, you're likely to get a spoonful of **Creamy Coleslaw** and maybe some of my **Big Bunch of Potato Salad.** On a breezy fall eve, I might offer **Italian Fried Potatoes** and **Green Bean Succotash.** And if you're invited for a festive spring luncheon, you might be find some **Carrot-Raisin Relish** and **Easy Macaroni Salad** decorating your plate. No matter the season or locale, you won't need a special reason to stir up these splendid sides!

Quick Side Dishes

Apple Cabin Salad

I stirred up this delicious blend when we were touring the magnificent Pacific Northwest, where the apples are the biggest anywhere! There's something irresistible about the mix of fruit and cheese, isn't there?   ♥   Serves 6 (full ¾ cup)

 ¼ cup Kraft fat-free mayonnaise
 ½ cup Cool Whip Free
 2 cups (4 small) cored, unpeeled, and diced Red Delicious apples
 1 cup seedless green grapes
 ¾ cup finely chopped celery
 ⅓ cup (1½ ounces) shredded Kraft reduced-fat Cheddar cheese
 ¼ cup (1 ounce) chopped walnuts

In a large bowl, combine mayonnaise and Cool Whip Free. Add apples, grapes, and celery. Mix well to combine. Stir in Cheddar cheese and walnuts. Cover and refrigerate for at least 30 minutes. Gently stir again just before serving.

Each serving equals:

HE: 1 Fruit • ½ Protein • ⅓ Fat • ¼ Vegetable • 17 Optional Calories

112 Calories • 4 gm Fat • 3 gm Protein • 16 gm Carbohydrate • 163 mg Sodium • 63 mg Calcium • 1 gm Fiber

DIABETIC EXCHANGES: 1 Fruit • ½ Meat • ½ Fat

Pineapple-Orange Salad

I've been teased about cooking with Diet Mountain Dew, but I say, why not use the most flavorful ingredients I can find! In this citrusy combo, you get a summer day's worth of sunshine in every mouthful.

☻ Serves 8

2 (4-serving) packages JELL-O sugar-free orange gelatin ☆
¾ cup boiling water
2 cups Diet Mountain Dew ☆
1 (8-ounce) can crushed pineapple, packed in fruit juice, undrained
1 (11-ounce) can mandarin oranges, rinsed and drained
1 (4-serving) package JELL-O sugar-free instant vanilla pudding mix
⅔ cup Carnation Nonfat Dry Milk Powder
¾ cup Cool Whip Free

In a large bowl, combine 1 package dry gelatin and boiling water. Mix well to dissolve gelatin. Stir in 1 cup Diet Mountain Dew and undrained pineapple. Add mandarin oranges. Mix well to combine. Pour mixture into an 8-by-8-inch dish. Refrigerate until set, about 3 hours. In a medium bowl, combine dry pudding mix, remaining package dry gelatin, and dry milk powder. Add remaining 1 cup Diet Mountain Dew. Mix well using a wire whisk. Blend in Cool Whip Free. Spread mixture evenly over set gelatin mixture. Refrigerate for at least 15 minutes. Cut into 8 servings.

Each serving equals:

HE: ½ Fruit • ¼ Fat-Free Milk • ¼ Slider • 9 Optional Calories

84 Calories • 0 gm Fat • 4 gm Protein • 17 gm Carbohydrate • 262 mg Sodium • 77 mg Calcium • 0 gm Fiber

DIABETIC EXCHANGES: ½ Fruit • ½ Starch/Carbohydrate

Kraut Relish

Sometimes the secret to good cooking is taking something handy, like canned sauerkraut, and stirring in some bits and pieces of flavor to make a good thing even better. What a great accompaniment to any grilled meat, especially pork. ☻ Serves 6 (½ cup)

> 1 (16-ounce) can sauerkraut, well drained
> ½ cup finely chopped celery
> ½ cup finely chopped green bell pepper
> ½ cup finely chopped carrots
> ½ cup finely chopped onion
> ¼ cup Splenda Granular

In a large bowl, combine sauerkraut, celery, green pepper, carrots, and onion. Add Splenda. Mix well to combine. Cover and refrigerate for at least 8 hours or overnight. Gently stir again just before serving.

Each serving equals:

HE: 1 Vegetable • 4 Optional Calories

28 Calories • 0 gm Fat • 1 gm Protein •
6 gm Carbohydrate • 532 mg Sodium •
34 mg Calcium • 3 gm Fiber

DIABETIC EXCHANGES: 1 Vegetable

Tomato Cucumber Relish

When Cliff and I set out on a summer road trip, we take some of the fresh bounty from my Iowa garden. This fresher-than-fresh salad is crisp and crunchy with just a touch of sweetness.

♥   Serves 8 (½ cup)

> 2 cups diced fresh tomatoes
> 1½ cups diced unpeeled cucumbers
> ½ cup diced onion
> ½ cup Kraft Fat Free Italian Dressing
> 1 tablespoon Splenda Granular

In a medium bowl, combine tomatoes, cucumbers, and onion. Add Italian dressing and Splenda. Mix gently to combine. Cover and refrigerate for at least 30 minutes. Gently stir again just before serving.

Each serving equals:

HE: 1 Vegetable • 12 Optional Calories

---

24 Calories • 0 gm Fat • 1 gm Protein •
5 gm Carbohydrate • 270 mg Sodium • 7 mg Calcium •
1 gm Fiber

DIABETIC EXCHANGES: 1 Vegetable

Carrot-Raisin Relish

Most of us can't afford a fancy salad shredder when we're traveling the highways and byways, so for a recipe like this one, we happily use convenient pre-cut veggies from the store. What a satisfying sweet-and-crunchy dish this is! ♥ Serves 6 (½ cup)

3 cups shredded carrots
¾ cup raisins
½ cup Kraft fat-free mayonnaise
2 tablespoons fat-free milk
1 tablespoon Splenda Granular
2 teaspoons lemon juice

In a large bowl, combine carrots and raisins. In a small bowl, combine mayonnaise, milk, Splenda, and lemon juice. Add mayonnaise mixture to carrot mixture. Mix well to combine. Cover and refrigerate for at least 30 minutes. Gently stir again just before serving.

Each serving equals:

HE: 1 Fruit • 1 Vegetable • 16 Optional Calories

96 Calories • 0 gm Fat • 1 gm Protein •
23 gm Carbohydrate • 197 mg Sodium •
30 mg Calcium • 2 gm Fiber

DIABETIC EXCHANGES: 1 Fruit • 1 Vegetable

French Corn Relish

As long as I have a couple of cans of corn in the pantry, I've got the makings of a tasty relish that won't lose its pizazz in the fridge.

❍ Serves 4 (½ cup)

1 (16-ounce) can whole-kernel corn, rinsed and drained
½ cup chopped onion
½ cup chopped green bell pepper
1 (2-ounce) jar chopped pimiento, drained
⅓ cup Kraft Fat Free French Dressing
1 teaspoon dried parsley flakes

In a large bowl, combine corn, onion, green pepper, and pimiento. Add French dressing and parsley flakes. Mix well to combine. Cover and refrigerate for at least 1 hour. Gently stir again just before serving.

Each serving equals:

HE: 1 Bread • ½ Vegetable • ¼ Slider •
13 Optional Calories

121 Calories • 1 gm Fat • 2 gm Protein •
26 gm Carbohydrate • 541 mg Sodium •
7 mg Calcium • 3 gm Fiber

DIABETIC EXCHANGES: 1½ Starch/Carbohydrate

Creamy Coleslaw

You can buy the same tired coleslaw in almost any takeout shop coast to coast, but why should you? Here's a quick and easy version that you can fix in a flash—and it tastes like the real thing!

◑ Serves 4 (1 cup)

½ cup Kraft fat-free mayonnaise
1½ tablespoons cider vinegar
2 tablespoons Splenda Granular
4 cups shredded cabbage

In a large bowl, combine mayonnaise, vinegar, and Splenda. Add cabbage. Mix well to combine. Cover and refrigerate for at least 1 hour. Gently stir again just before serving.

Each serving equals:

HE: 1 Vegetable • ¼ Slider • 3 Optional Calories

40 Calories • 0 gm Fat • 1 gm Protein •
9 gm Carbohydrate • 273 mg Sodium •
33 mg Calcium • 1 gm Fiber

DIABETIC EXCHANGES: 1 Vegetable

Hawaiian Ham Pasta Salad

Here's a dish with a wonderful blend of tastes and textures, perfect for a quick lunch at a roadside table. Even if Maui isn't on the map this time around, you can relish the flavors of the islands.

⭕ Serves 4 (1¼ cups)

> 1½ cups (9 ounces) finely chopped Dubuque 97% fat-free ham or any extra-lean ham
> 1 (8-ounce) can pineapple tidbits, packed in fruit juice, drained and ¼ cup liquid reserved
> 2 cups cold cooked rotini pasta, rinsed and drained
> ¾ cup diced celery
> ¼ cup chopped green onion
> ⅓ cup Kraft fat-free mayonnaise

In a large bowl, combine ham, pineapple, pasta, celery, and onion. In a medium bowl, combine mayonnaise and reserved pineapple juice. Add dressing mixture to pasta mixture. Mix well to combine. Cover and refrigerate for at least 30 minutes. Gently stir again just before serving.

HINT: Usually 1½ cups uncooked rotini pasta cooks to about 2 cups.

Each serving equals:

HE: 1½ Protein • 1 Bread • ½ Fruit • ½ Vegetable • 13 Optional Calories

194 Calories • 2 gm Fat • 14 gm Protein •
30 gm Carbohydrate • 695 mg Sodium •
22 mg Calcium • 2 gm Fiber

DIABETIC EXCHANGES: 1½ Meat • 1 Starch • ½ Fruit •
½ Vegetable

Easy Macaroni Salad

This dish works best when the macaroni is prepared in advance and chilled in your refrigerator. Make it in the morning for an evening meal, or the night before if you're planning to serve it for lunch the next day.   ○   Serves 4 (¾ cup)

> 2 cups cold cooked elbow macaroni, rinsed and drained
> ¾ cup shredded carrots
> ¼ cup chopped green onion
> ½ cup Kraft fat-free mayonnaise
> 2 tablespoons Land O Lakes no-fat sour cream
> 1 teaspoon dried parsley flakes
> ½ teaspoon prepared yellow mustard

In a medium bowl, combine macaroni, carrots, and green onion. Add mayonnaise, sour cream, parsley flakes, and mustard. Mix well to combine. Cover and refrigerate for at least 30 minutes. Gently stir again just before serving.

HINT: Usually 1⅓ cups uncooked elbow macaroni cooks to about 2 cups.

Each serving equals:

HE: 1 Bread • ½ Vegetable • ¼ Slider • 8 Optional Calories

128 Calories • 0 gm Fat • 4 gm Protein • 28 gm Carbohydrate • 286 mg Sodium • 22 mg Calcium • 2 gm Fiber

DIABETIC EXCHANGES: 1½ Starch • ½ Vegetable

A Big Bunch of Potato Salad

Cooking for a crowd? Here's a recipe that can star at a picnic or a summer supper for family and friends. You can cook the potatoes ahead and have all the ingredients ready, so that preparation is easy as pie. (You'll even have time to make a pie!)

◐ Serves 12 (scant 1 cup)

> 7 full cups (36 ounces) diced cooked potatoes
> 1 cup chopped onion
> 2 cups chopped celery
> 2 cups Kraft fat-free mayonnaise
> 2 tablespoons Splenda Granular
> 2 tablespoons fat-free milk
> ⅓ cup sweet pickle relish
> 1 tablespoon prepared yellow mustard
> 6 hard-boiled eggs, chopped

In a very large bowl, combine potatoes, onion, and celery. In a medium bowl, combine mayonnaise, Splenda, milk, pickle relish, and mustard. Add dressing mixture to potato mixture. Mix gently to combine. Fold in chopped eggs. Cover and refrigerate for at least 1 hour. Gently stir again just before serving.

Each serving equals:

HE: ¾ Bread • ½ Protein • ½ Vegetable • ¼ Slider • 16 Optional Calories

159 Calories • 3 gm Fat • 5 gm Protein • 28 gm Carbohydrate • 469 mg Sodium • 32 mg Calcium • 2 gm Fiber

DIABETIC EXCHANGES: 1 Starch • ½ Meat • ½ Vegetable

Old-fashioned Potato Salad

I've created so many potato salads over the years, but each time I decide to try again, I find new pleasure in a fresh combination. I hope this version wins a spot on your Top Ten List of favorites!

⚫ Serves 6 (1 cup)

1 cup Kraft fat-free mayonnaise
2 tablespoons white distilled vinegar
1 tablespoon Splenda Granular
1 teaspoon dried parsley flakes
5 cups (24 ounces) diced cooked potatoes
1 cup chopped celery
½ cup chopped onion
2 hard-boiled eggs, chopped

In a large bowl, combine mayonnaise, vinegar, Splenda, and parsley flakes. Add potatoes, celery, and onion. Mix well to combine. Fold in chopped eggs. Cover and refrigerate for at least 1 hour. Gently stir again just before serving.

Each serving equals:

HE: 1 Bread • ½ Vegetable • ⅓ Protein • ¼ Slider • 9 Optional Calories

166 Calories • 2 gm Fat • 5 gm Protein • 32 gm Carbohydrate • 399 mg Sodium • 25 mg Calcium • 3 gm Fiber

DIABETIC EXCHANGES: 1½ Starch • ½ Vegetable

Southern Vegetable Skillet

They like their vegetables sweeter down South than almost anywhere else, so I created this recipe with southern palates in mind. There's plenty of natural sweetness in veggies like carrots and corn, anyway, so this skillet sensation makes perfect sense.

◐ Serves 4 (1 cup)

> 2 cups sliced unpeeled zucchini
> ½ cup chopped onion
> 1 cup shredded carrots
> 1 (16-ounce) can whole-kernel corn, rinsed and drained
> 1½ cups reduced-sodium tomato juice
> 2 tablespoons Splenda Granular
> 1 teaspoon dried parsley flakes

In a large skillet sprayed with butter-flavored cooking spray, sauté zucchini, onion, and carrots for 5 minutes or until just tender. Add corn, tomato juice, Splenda, and parsley flakes. Mix gently to combine. Lower heat, cover, and simmer for 10 minutes, stirring occasionally.

Each serving equals:

HE: 2½ Vegetable • 1 Bread • 3 Optional Calories

124 Calories • 0 gm Fat • 4 gm Protein •
27 gm Carbohydrate • 26 mg Sodium •
33 mg Calcium • 5 gm Fiber

DIABETIC EXCHANGES: 2 Vegetable • 1 Starch

Layered Tomato Casserole

Depending on where the map takes you, you should be able to get good tomatoes all year long. Even in the cold months, this recipe will make a great tomato taste even better, and a so-so tomato deserve four stars!   ☉   Serves 6

5½ cups peeled and sliced fresh tomatoes ☆
½ cup chopped onion ☆
1 cup + 2 tablespoons (4½ ounces) shredded Kraft reduced-fat
   Cheddar cheese ☆
20 Ritz Reduced Fat Crackers, made into crumbs ☆
¼ cup Kraft Fat Free Thousand Island Dressing

Preheat oven to 350 degrees. Spray an 8-by-8-inch baking dish with butter-flavored cooking spray. Layer half of tomatoes, half of onion, half of Cheddar cheese, and half of cracker crumbs in prepared baking dish. Repeat layers with tomatoes, onion, and Cheddar cheese. Evenly spoon Thousand Island dressing over Cheddar cheese. Sprinkle remaining cracker crumbs over top. Bake for 45 to 50 minutes. Place baking dish on a wire rack and let set for 5 minutes. Cut into 6 servings.

HINT: A self-seal sandwich bag works great for crushing crackers.

Each serving equals:

HE: 1 Vegetable • 1 Protein • ⅔ Bread •
17 Optional Calories

149 Calories • 5 gm Fat • 7 gm Protein •
19 gm Carbohydrate • 377 mg Sodium •
162 mg Calcium • 2 gm Fiber

DIABETIC EXCHANGES: 1 Vegetable • 1 Meat • 1 Starch

Please Pass the Peas Side Dish

Tiny peas arrive with a special flavor all their own, but you'll discover with pleasure how a quick sauté with a piquant salad dressing can work some culinary magic. Just remember to say "please" when you are ready for seconds!   ☻   Serves 4 (full ½ cup)

½ cup finely chopped onion
1 (16-ounce) can tiny peas, rinsed and drained
1 (2.5-ounce) jar sliced mushrooms, drained
½ cup Kraft Fat Free Honey Dijon Salad Dressing

In a large skillet sprayed with butter-flavored cooking spray, sauté onion for 5 minutes or until tender. Stir in peas and mushrooms. Add Honey Dijon dressing. Mix well to combine. Lower heat and simmer for 5 minutes or until mixture is heated through, stirring often.

Each serving equals:

HE: 1 Bread • ½ Vegetable • ½ Slider •
10 Optional Calories

128 Calories • 0 gm Fat • 4 gm Protein •
28 gm Carbohydrate • 357 mg Sodium •
24 mg Calcium • 5 gm Fiber

DIABETIC EXCHANGES: 1½ Starch/Carbohydrate •
½ Vegetable

Unbelievably Good Green Beans

If Cliff is in the driver's seat (and he almost always is!), then I need plenty of green bean recipes to serve along the way. This one finds its inspiration in a classic Caesar salad, with just enough Parmesan cheese to make it truly tangy!   ❍   Serves 4 (1 cup)

½ cup finely chopped onion
2 (16-ounce) cans cut green beans, rinsed and drained
1 (2-ounce) jar chopped pimiento, undrained
½ cup Kraft Classic Caesar Dressing
¼ cup (¾ ounce) Kraft Reduced Fat Parmesan Style Grated
    Topping
2 tablespoons Hormel Bacon Bits

In a large skillet sprayed with butter-flavored cooking spray, sauté onion for 5 minutes. Stir in green beans and undrained pimiento. Add Caesar dressing, Parmesan cheese, and bacon bits. Mix well to combine. Lower heat and simmer for 5 minutes, stirring often.

Each serving equals:

HE: 1¼ Vegetable • ¼ Protein • ¾ Slider •
3 Optional Calories

122 Calories • 6 gm Fat • 4 gm Protein •
13 gm Carbohydrate • 537 mg Sodium •
30 mg Calcium • 2 gm Fiber

DIABETIC EXCHANGES: 1½ Vegetable •
½ Starch/Carbohydrate • ½ Fat

Simmered Green Beans

Make sure you replace your spices every six months to a year, especially when you notice a change in their color. Dried basil adds so much to these green beans, but this delectable ingredient can't do its stuff if it's been sitting on your shelf for years.

○ Serves 4 (1 cup)

> ½ cup chopped onion
> 4 cups frozen cut green beans, thawed
> 1 teaspoon dried basil leaves
> 1 tablespoon Splenda Granular
> ⅛ teaspoon black pepper
> ¼ cup boiling water

In a large skillet sprayed with olive oil–flavored cooking spray, sauté onion for 5 minutes. Add green beans, basil, Splenda, black pepper, and water. Cover and simmer for 15 minutes, stirring occasionally.

HINT: Thaw green beans by placing in a colander and rinsing under hot water for 1 minute.

Each serving equals:

HE: 2 Vegetable • 1 Optional Calorie

60 Calories • 0 gm Fat • 3 gm Protein •
12 gm Carbohydrate • 5 mg Sodium • 69 mg Calcium •
4 gm Fiber

DIABETIC EXCHANGES: 2 Vegetable

Green Bean Succotash

Corn and beans are two truly all-American vegetables, and together they prove just how much better we can be when we work together toward a goal. In this case, it's the side dish that turns any old meal into a celebration. ☺ Serves 4 (¾ cup)

1 (16-ounce) can whole-kernel corn, rinsed and drained
1 (16-ounce) can cut green beans, rinsed and drained
2 teaspoons I Can't Believe It's Not Butter! Light Margarine
⅓ cup Carnation Nonfat Dry Milk Powder
⅓ cup water
⅛ teaspoon black pepper

In a medium saucepan, combine corn, green beans, and margarine. Cook over medium heat until mixture is heated through, stirring often. In a small bowl, combine dry milk powder, water, and black pepper. Add milk mixture to vegetable mixture. Mix well to combine. Continue cooking for about 2 to 3 minutes, stirring often.

Each serving equals:

HE: 1 Bread • 1 Vegetable • ¼ Fat-Free Milk • ¼ Fat

122 Calories • 2 gm Fat • 5 gm Protein •
21 gm Carbohydrate • 603 mg Sodium •
95 mg Calcium • 4 gm Fiber

DIABETIC EXCHANGES: 1 Starch • 1 Vegetable

Green Bean and Bacon Bake

"Simply scrumptious" was the echo I heard when I asked family members to tell me honestly what they thought of this cheesy, creamy, baked veggie dish. I think Cliff could eat this once a week for a year if I made it for him!   ◐   Serves 6

> 15 Ritz Reduced Fat Crackers, made into crumbs ☆
> 2 (16-ounce) cans cut green beans, rinsed and drained ☆
> ½ cup finely chopped onion ☆
> 1 (10¾-ounce) can Healthy Request Cream of Mushroom Soup ☆
> ¾ cup (3 ounces) shredded Kraft reduced-fat Cheddar cheese
> ¼ cup Hormel Bacon Bits

Preheat oven to 350 degrees. Spray an 8-by-8-inch baking dish with butter-flavored cooking spray. Layer half of cracker crumbs, half of green beans, and half of onion in prepared baking dish. Spoon half of mushroom soup over top. Layer Cheddar cheese, remaining green beans, and remaining onion over top. Spoon remaining mushroom soup over all. Sprinkle remaining cracker crumbs and bacon bits over soup. Lightly spray top with butter-flavored cooking spray. Bake for 30 to 35 minutes. Place baking dish on a wire rack and let set for 5 minutes. Divide into 6 servings.

HINT: A self-seal sandwich bag works great for crushing crackers.

Each serving equals:

HE: 1½ Vegetable • ⅔ Protein • ½ Bread • ½ Slider • 4 Optional Calories

137 Calories • 5 gm Fat • 8 gm Protein • 15 gm Carbohydrate • 803 mg Sodium • 169 mg Calcium • 3 gm Fiber

DIABETIC EXCHANGES: 1½ Vegetable • 1 Meat • ½ Starch

Carrots Olé

Cliff loves all kinds of salsa, the hotter the better, so when we travel, we often try a regional brand or two, just to taste the difference. This delectable carrot dish is ideal for doing just that!

☻ Serves 4 (½ cup)

3 cups shredded carrots
2 cups hot water
1 teaspoon dried parsley flakes
½ cup chunky salsa (mild, medium, or hot)
2 tablespoons Hormel Bacon Bits

In a medium saucepan, cook carrots in water for 10 minutes or until just tender. Drain and return carrots to saucepan. Add parsley flakes, salsa, and bacon bits. Mix well to combine. Continue cooking until heated through, stirring often.

Each serving equals:

HE: 1¾ Vegetable • 12 Optional Calories

---

57 Calories • 1 gm Fat • 2 gm Protein •
10 gm Carbohydrate • 264 mg Sodium •
64 mg Calcium • 2 gm Fiber

DIABETIC EXCHANGES: 2 Vegetable

Swiss Simmered Carrots

Some people believe that fresh is always better than anything else, but frozen veggies are a terrific alternative. These carrots are sliced just after picking and kept just right til you're ready to cook 'em up. Use any canned tomatoes you like, including those with yummy extras like green chiles.　❂　Serves 6 (⅔ cup)

> 1 cup chopped celery
> 1 cup chopped onion
> 1 (10¾-ounce) can Healthy Request Tomato Soup
> 1 (8-ounce) can tomatoes, chopped and undrained
> 1 tablespoon Splenda Granular
> 1 teaspoon dried parsley flakes
> ⅛ teaspoon black pepper
> 3 cups frozen sliced carrots, thawed

In a large skillet sprayed with butter-flavored cooking spray, sauté celery and onion for 5 minutes. Stir in tomato soup, undrained tomatoes, Splenda, parsley flakes, and black pepper. Add carrots. Mix well to combine. Lower heat, cover, and simmer for 25 to 30 minutes or until vegetables are tender, stirring occasionally.

HINT: Thaw carrots by placing in a colander and rinsing under hot water for 1 minute.

Each serving equals:

HE: 2 Vegetable • ¼ Slider • 11 Optional Calories

---

77 Calories • 1 gm Fat • 1 gm Protein •
16 gm Carbohydrate • 308 mg Sodium •
34 mg Calcium • 3 gm Fiber

DIABETIC EXCHANGES: 2 Vegetable

Carrot Casserole

Sometimes it's the side dish that makes the meal special, and this one is a scrumptious surprise from the very first bite. Cheese and carrots are a winning combination every time! ○ Serves 6

2 (16-ounce) cans sliced carrots, rinsed and drained
1 (10¾-ounce) can Healthy Request Cream of Celery or Mushroom
    Soup
¾ cup (3 ounces) shredded Kraft reduced-fat Cheddar cheese
6 tablespoons dried fine bread crumbs

Preheat oven to 350 degrees. Spray an 8-by-8-inch baking dish with butter-flavored cooking spray. In a large bowl, combine carrots, celery soup, and Cheddar cheese. Spread mixture into prepared baking dish. Evenly sprinkle bread crumbs over top. Lightly spray bread crumbs with butter-flavored cooking spray. Bake for 25 to 30 minutes. Place baking dish on a wire rack and let set for 5 minutes. Divide into 6 servings.

Each serving equals:

HE: 1⅓ Vegetable • ⅔ Protein • ⅓ Bread • ¼ Slider •
8 Optional Calories

128 Calories • 4 gm Fat • 6 gm Protein •
17 gm Carbohydrate • 607 mg Sodium •
176 mg Calcium • 3 gm Fiber

DIABETIC EXCHANGES: 1 Vegetable • ½ Meat • ½ Starch

Macaroni Stroganoff

Can a recipe really be this creamy and not be brimming over with unhealthy fat? The answer is a resounding "Yes!" So—invite your guests to partake with pleasure of this luscious macaroni mix.

○ Serves 6 (⅔ cup)

> ½ cup finely chopped onion
> ½ cup chopped celery
> 1 (10¾-ounce) can Healthy Request Cream of Mushroom Soup
> ½ cup Land O Lakes no-fat sour cream
> ⅛ teaspoon black pepper
> 2 (2.5-ounce) jars sliced mushrooms, drained
> 1 (8-ounce) can tiny peas, rinsed and drained
> 2 cups hot cooked elbow macaroni, rinsed and drained

In a large skillet sprayed with butter-flavored cooking spray, sauté onion and celery for 6 to 8 minutes. Stir in mushroom soup, sour cream, and black pepper. Add mushrooms and peas. Mix well to combine. Fold in macaroni. Lower heat and simmer for 6 to 8 minutes or until mixture is heated through, stirring occasionally.

HINT: Usually 1⅓ cups uncooked elbow macaroni cooks to about 2 cups.

Each serving equals:

> HE: 1 Bread • ⅔ Vegetable • ½ Slider •
> 8 Optional Calories
>
> ---
> 150 Calories • 2 gm Fat • 5 gm Protein •
> 28 gm Carbohydrate • 338 mg Sodium •
> 68 mg Calcium • 3 gm Fiber
>
> ---
> DIABETIC EXCHANGES: 1½ Starch/Carbohydrate •
> ½ Vegetable

Mushroom Rice Side Dish

It's a smart cook's secret—cooking rice in a liquid more flavorful than plain old water. Broth is good, and this spice-and-soup combo is better still, for a dish that will make everyone at the table applaud the cook! ☻ Serves 6 (⅔ cup)

> 1 (14½-ounce) can Swanson Beef Broth
> 1 (10¾-ounce) can Healthy Request Cream of Mushroom Soup
> 2 teaspoons dried onion flakes
> 1 teaspoon dried parsley flakes
> 2 (2.5-ounce) jars sliced mushrooms, drained
> 1⅓ cups (4 ounces) uncooked Minute Rice

In a large skillet, combine beef broth, mushroom soup, onion flakes, and parsley flakes. Stir in mushrooms. Bring mixture to a boil. Add uncooked rice. Mix well to combine. Lower heat, cover, and simmer for 10 minutes or until rice is tender, stirring occasionally.

HINT: Great with hamburger or roast beef.

Each serving equals:

HE: ⅔ Bread • ⅓ Vegetable • ¼ Slider •
13 Optional Calories

73 Calories • 1 gm Fat • 2 gm Protein •
14 gm Carbohydrate • 551 mg Sodium •
41 mg Calcium • 1 gm Fiber

DIABETIC EXCHANGES: 1 Starch

Lone Star Scalloped Potatoes

With a flavor as big as the state President Bush calls home, this luscious potato dish is almost a meal in itself. When you've got the time, they've got the taste! ☯ Serves 4

1½ cups (6 ounces) diced Velveeta Light processed cheese
½ cup chunky salsa (mild, medium, or hot)
4 cups (20 ounces) thinly sliced raw potatoes
1 teaspoon dried parsley flakes

Preheat oven to 350 degrees. Spray an 8-by-8-inch baking dish with olive oil–flavored cooking spray. In a large saucepan, combine cheese and salsa. Cook over medium heat until cheese melts, stirring often. Add potatoes and parsley flakes. Mix well to combine. Spread mixture into prepared baking dish. Cover and bake for 60 minutes or until potatoes are tender. Uncover and place baking dish on a wire rack and let set for 5 minutes. Divide into 4 servings.

Each serving equals:

HE: 2 Protein • 1 Bread • ¼ Vegetable

225 Calories • 5 gm Fat • 12 gm Protein •
33 gm Carbohydrate • 803 mg Sodium •
255 mg Calcium • 3 gm Fiber

DIABETIC EXCHANGES: 1½ Meat • 1 Starch

Italian Fried Potatoes

I don't know if the creators of my favorite bottled Italian dressing had any idea what lengths I'd go to with their creation, but once you've bathed plain old potatoes in it, you'll be ready to hum, "That's *Amore!*"   ☻   Serves 4 (¾ cup)

¼ *cup Kraft Fat Free Italian Dressing*
½ *cup chopped onion*
3 *cups (15 ounces) sliced raw potatoes*

Pour Italian dressing in a large skillet. Cook over medium heat until hot. Add onion and potatoes. Mix well to combine. Cover and cook for about 15 to 20 minutes or until tender. Uncover and continue cooking until potatoes are browned, stirring occasionally.

Each serving equals:

HE: ¾ Bread • ¼ Vegetable • 8 Optional Calories

76 Calories • 0 gm Fat • 2 gm Protein •
17 gm Carbohydrate • 161 mg Sodium •
11 mg Calcium • 2 gm Fiber

DIABETIC EXCHANGES: 1 Starch

Fast Main Dishes

When you're on the road, the last thing you want to do is spend hours fixing complicated meals—but you've got to eat, don't you? And while it's fun to try the regional cuisine or tasty road food as you pass through small towns and big cities, you're likely to choose a "home-cooked" meal much of the time. Sometimes it's because a taste of home provides a special comfort when you're far away; other times, it's because nothing tastes as good as a savory meat loaf when it's prepared with love. After a couple of weeks on book tour, all Cliff wants is a comfy Healthy Exchanges skillet supper—and green beans made my way!

If you're looking for entrees that don't taste as if you rushed, you've come to the right place! Whether you're longing for comfort food with a little sizzle (**South of the Border Macaroni and Cheese** will fit the bill) or hungry for something lusciously creamy (choose **Country Stroganoff with Rice** or **Layered Scalloped Potatoes and Ham**), you won't have to choose between healthy and delicious. And if you've only got time for a meal on the run, you can opt for **Hot Dog Wraps** or **Salmon Burgers!**

Fast Main Dishes

Creole Campfire Fish

There's a special smoky goodness to the dishes we cook over a campfire, don't you think? Here, I've tried to duplicate that out-in-the-woods taste with a bit of culinary magic, and you don't even have to gather a stick of wood! ☻ Serves 4

¼ cup chopped green bell pepper
¾ cup chopped onion
1 (8-ounce) can Hunt's Tomato Sauce
1 tablespoon Worcestershire sauce
16 ounces white fish, cut into 4 pieces

Cut four (18-inch) pieces of heavy duty aluminum foil. In a medium skillet sprayed with butter-flavored cooking spray, sauté green pepper and onion for 5 minutes or until tender. Add tomato sauce and Worcestershire sauce. Mix well to combine. Place one piece of fish in center of each piece of foil. Lightly spray each with butter-flavored cooking spray. Drizzle ¼ cup sauce over top of each. Wrap and double seal. Place on grill and cook for 15 to 20 minutes, turning occasionally.

HINT: If desired, packets could be placed on a large baking sheet and baked at 350 degrees for 30 minutes, turning occasionally.

Each serving equals:

HE: 2½ Protein • 1½ Vegetable

186 Calories • 6 gm Fat • 25 gm Protein •
8 gm Carbohydrate • 445 mg Sodium •
49 mg Calcium • 1 gm Fiber

DIABETIC EXCHANGES: 3 Meat • 1 Vegetable

Quick Tuna Casserole

Even if you've got a recipe box filled with tuna noodle casserole recipes, I hope you'll give this speedy version a try. It's as fast as it is flavorful, and it's also a great money saver when you're feeding a large family.   ☺   Serves 6

⅔ cup Carnation Nonfat Dry Milk Powder
¾ cup water
1 (10¾-ounce) can Healthy Request Cream of Mushroom Soup
2 tablespoons dried onion flakes
1 teaspoon dried parsley flakes
2½ cups hot cooked noodles, rinsed and drained
2 (6-ounce) cans white tuna, packed in water, drained and flaked
½ cup (¾ ounce) crushed cornflakes

Preheat oven to 350 degrees. Spray an 8-by-8-inch baking dish with butter-flavored cooking spray. In a medium bowl, combine dry milk powder and water. Add mushroom soup, onion flakes, and parsley flakes. Mix well to combine. Stir in noodles and tuna. Pour mixture into prepared baking dish. Evenly sprinkle cornflake crumbs over top. Bake for 25 to 30 minutes. Place baking dish on a wire rack and let set for 5 minutes. Divide into 6 servings.

HINT: Usually 2 cups uncooked noodles cooks to about 2½ cups.

Each serving equals:

HE: 1½ Protein • 1 Bread • ⅓ Fat-Free Milk •
¼ Slider • 8 Optional Calories

219 Calories • 3 gm Fat • 21 gm Protein •
27 gm Carbohydrate • 459 mg Sodium •
144 mg Calcium • 1 gm Fiber

DIABETIC EXCHANGES: 2 Meat • 1½ Starch/Carbohydrate

Easy Creamed Tuna

Back in the 1950s, creamy tuna dishes appeared on every mom's list of favorite lunchtime dishes. If you're in the mood for a bit of time travel back to those good old days, try this warm and wonderful recipe soon.   ☺   Serves 4 (⅔ cup)

½ cup chopped onion
1 (10¾-ounce) can Healthy Request Cream of Celery Soup
⅓ cup Carnation Nonfat Dry Milk Powder
⅓ cup water
1 (2.5-ounce) jar sliced mushrooms, drained
1 (6-ounce) can white tuna, packed in water, drained and flaked
1 (2-ounce) jar chopped pimiento, undrained
2 teaspoons dried parsley flakes

In a large skillet sprayed with butter-flavored cooking spray, sauté onion for 5 minutes. In a medium bowl, combine celery soup, dry milk powder, and water. Stir soup mixture into skillet. Add mushrooms, tuna, undrained pimiento, and parsley flakes. Mix well to combine. Lower heat and simmer for 5 minutes, stirring occasionally.

HINT: Good over toast, rice, or potatoes.

Each serving equals:

HE: 1 Protein • ½ Vegetable • ¼ Fat-Free Milk • ½ Slider • 1 Optional Calorie

127 Calories • 3 gm Fat • 13 gm Protein • 12 gm Carbohydrate • 565 mg Sodium • 151 mg Calcium • 1 gm Fiber

DIABETIC EXCHANGES: 1½ Meat • ½ Starch/Carbohydrate • ½ Vegetable

Speedy Macaroni and Cheese with Tuna Skillet

When everyone is too hungry to wait, this is just the right meal to serve up in seconds! It tastes of home when you're miles and miles away, and that's got to be good.   ◑   Serves 4 (1 cup)

1 (10¾-ounce) can Healthy Request Cream of Mushroom Soup
⅓ cup fat-free milk
1½ cups (6 ounces) shredded Kraft reduced-fat Cheddar cheese
1 teaspoon dried onion flakes
1 teaspoon dried parsley flakes
⅛ teaspoon black pepper
1 (6-ounce) can white tuna, packed in water, drained and flaked
2 cups cooked hot elbow macaroni, rinsed and drained

In a large skillet, combine mushroom soup, milk, and Cheddar cheese. Cook over medium heat, until cheese starts to melt, stirring often. Add onion flakes, parsley flakes, black pepper, and tuna. Mix well to combine. Stir in macaroni. Lower heat and simmer for 5 minutes, stirring occasionally.

HINT: Usually 1⅓ cups uncooked elbow macaroni cooks to about 2 cups.

Each serving equals:

HE: 3 Protein • 1 Bread • ½ Slider • 9 Optional Calories

297 Calories • 9 gm Fat • 28 gm Protein • 26 gm Carbohydrate • 805 mg Sodium • 380 mg Calcium • 1 gm Fiber

DIABETIC EXCHANGES: 3 Meat • 1½ Starch

Pasta with Tuna Sauce

There's a famous Italian veal dish served with a sauce of tuna, and it's always intrigued me. I decided to make the tuna the star of this pasta meal, and to combine it with creamy, cheesy flavors that warm the heart and tummy all at once.   ☺   Serves 4 (1 cup)

> 1 (6-ounce) can white tuna, packed in water, drained and flaked
> 2 cups peeled and chopped fresh tomatoes
> ½ teaspoon dried minced garlic
> 1 tablespoon chopped fresh parsley or 1 teaspoon dried
> parsley flakes
> ⅛ teaspoon black pepper
> 1 teaspoon Italian seasoning
> 1 (10¾-ounce) can Healthy Request Cream of Mushroom Soup
> 2 cups hot, cooked spaghetti, rinsed and drained
> ¼ cup (¾ ounce) Kraft Reduced Fat Parmesan Style Grated
> Topping

In a large skillet sprayed with olive oil–flavored cooking spray, sauté tuna, tomatoes, garlic, parsley, black pepper, and Italian seasoning. Cook over medium-low heat for about 10 minutes or until tomatoes are tender and mixture is slightly thickened, stirring often. Stir in mushroom soup. Add spaghetti and Parmesan cheese. Mix well to combine. Lower heat and simmer for 5 minutes or until mixture is heated through, stirring often.

HINT: Usually 1½ cups broken uncooked spaghetti cooks to about 2 cups.

Each serving equals:

> HE: 1¾ Protein • 1 Bread • 1 Vegetable • ½ Slider •
> 1 Optional Calorie
>
> ───
> 219 Calories • 3 gm Fat • 16 gm Protein •
> 32 gm Carbohydrate • 545 mg Sodium •
> 84 mg Calcium • 4 gm Fiber
> ───
> DIABETIC EXCHANGES: 2 Meat •
> 1½ Starch/Carbohydrate • 1 Vegetable

Quick Tuna Tetrazzini

With a well-stocked fridge and cabinets lined with handy canned goods, you're ready to make this dish quicker than you can say, E-Z Pass! We've figured out ways to make travel fast and easy, why not try those techniques in the kitchen as well?   ○   Serves 4 (1 cup)

> 1 (10¾-ounce) can Healthy Request Cream of Mushroom Soup
> 1 (9¼-ounce) can white tuna, packed in water, drained and flaked
> 1 teaspoon dried parsley flakes
> 1 (2-ounce) jar chopped pimiento, undrained
> ⅓ cup (1½ ounces) shredded Kraft reduced-fat Cheddar cheese
> ¼ cup fat-free milk
> 2 cups hot cooked spaghetti, rinsed and drained

In a large skillet sprayed with butter-flavored cooking spray, combine mushroom soup, tuna, parsley flakes, undrained pimiento, Cheddar cheese, and milk. Add spaghetti. Mix well to combine. Cook over medium heat until mixture is heated through and cheese is melted, stirring often.

HINT: Usually 1½ cups broken uncooked spaghetti cooks to about 2 cups.

Each serving equals:

HE: 2 Protein • 1 Bread • ½ Slider •
7 Optional Calories

---

250 Calories • 6 gm Fat • 22 gm Protein •
27 gm Carbohydrate • 651 mg Sodium •
156 mg Calcium • 1 gm Fiber

DIABETIC EXCHANGES: 2½ Meat • 1½ Starch

Celery Salmon Loaf

Salmon loaf was very popular a few decades back, when thrifty home cooks prepared it for their families as a special treat. It's still a scrumptious option, a way to transform canned fish into an entree that is hearty and light all at once. ☻ Serves 6

> 1 (10¾-ounce) can Healthy Request Cream of Celery Soup
> 1 egg or equivalent in egg substitute
> ¼ teaspoon lemon pepper
> 1 (14¾-ounce) can pink salmon, drained, boned, and flaked
> ¾ cup finely chopped celery
> ¼ cup finely chopped onion
> ¾ cup (3 ounces) dried fine bread crumbs

Preheat oven to 350 degrees. Spray a 9-by-5-inch loaf pan with butter-flavored cooking spray. In a large bowl, combine celery soup, egg, and lemon pepper. Add salmon, celery, onion, and bread crumbs. Mix well to combine. Pat mixture into prepared loaf pan. Bake for 55 to 60 minutes or until firm. Place loaf pan on a wire rack and let set for 5 minutes. Divide into 6 servings.

Each serving equals:

HE: 2 Protein • ⅔ Bread • ⅓ Vegetable • ¼ Slider • 8 Optional Calories

169 Calories • 5 gm Fat • 16 gm Protein • 15 gm Carbohydrate • 676 mg Sodium • 171 mg Calcium • 1 gm Fiber

DIABETIC EXCHANGES: 2½ Meat • 1 Starch

Salmon Burgers

If you can mold it into a patty, you can make it into a burger—and that's just what I did with some rich pink salmon! It's a wonderful change from the same old thing, and it's also a great healthy alternative to meat, meat, meat. ☺ Serves 6

1 (14¾-ounce) can pink salmon, drained, boned, and flaked
6 tablespoons (1½ ounces) dried fine bread crumbs
1 tablespoon dried onion flakes
1 tablespoon dried parsley flakes
⅓ cup reduced-sodium ketchup
⅓ cup (1½ ounces) shredded Kraft reduced-fat Cheddar cheese
1 egg or equivalent in egg substitute
1 teaspoon prepared yellow mustard
6 small hamburger buns

In a large bowl, combine salmon, bread crumbs, onion flakes, parsley flakes, ketchup, Cheddar cheese, egg, and mustard. Mix well to combine. Using a ⅓ cup measuring cup as a guide, form into 6 patties. Place patties in a large skillet sprayed with butter-flavored cooking spray. Brown patties for 3 minutes on each side or until golden brown. For each sandwich, place a patty between a hamburger bun. Serve at once.

Each serving equals:

HE: 2½ Protein • 1⅓ Bread • ⅔ Vegetable

244 Calories • 8 gm Fat • 20 gm Protein •
23 gm Carbohydrate • 687 mg Sodium •
223 mg Calcium • 1 gm Fiber

DIABETIC EXCHANGES: 3 Meat • 1½ Starch •
½ Vegetable

Bayou Country Creole Shrimp

You don't have to be motoring down a Louisiana highway in order to enjoy the flavors of one of my favorite cuisines! We've gotten wonderful shrimp at great prices from the warehouse stores, so shrimp doesn't have to be a special occasion food anymore.

○ Serves 6 (scant ¾ cup)

> 1 cup chopped onion
> 1 cup chopped green bell pepper
> 1 (10¾-ounce) can Healthy Request Tomato Soup
> 1 (8-ounce) can tomatoes, finely chopped and undrained
> 1 to 3 drops Tabasco sauce
> ⅛ teaspoon black pepper
> 1 teaspoon dried parsley flakes
> 1 (6-ounce) package frozen shelled shrimp, thawed
> 1½ cups hot cooked rice

In a large skillet sprayed with butter-flavored cooking spray, sauté onion and green pepper for 5 minutes. Stir in tomato soup, undrained tomatoes, Tabasco sauce, black pepper, and parsley flakes. Add shrimp and rice. Mix well to combine. Lower heat and simmer for 6 to 8 minutes, stirring occasionally.

HINT: Usually 1 cup uncooked instant rice cooks to about 1½ cups.

Each serving equals:

> HE: 1 Protein • 1 Vegetable • ½ Bread •
> 1 Optional Calorie
> ___
> 126 Calories • 2 gm Fat • 8 gm Protein •
> 19 gm Carbohydrate • 307 mg Sodium •
> 30 mg Calcium • 1 gm Fiber
> ___
> DIABETIC EXCHANGES: 1 Meat • 1 Vegetable • ½ Starch

Calico Chicken Tetrazzini

I've always liked dishes as appealing to the eye as they are to the taste buds, so I stirred lots of color and texture into this chicken-and-pasta combination. It's fun to find little surprises in each and every bite!

● Serves 4 (1 cup)

> 1½ cups (8 ounces) chopped cooked chicken breast
> ½ cup chopped red onion
> ½ cup chopped green bell pepper
> 1 (10¾-ounce) can Healthy Request Cream of Chicken Soup
> ¼ cup water
> 1 (2.5-ounce) jar sliced mushrooms, undrained
> 1 (2-ounce) jar chopped pimiento, undrained
> ¾ cup (3 ounces) shredded Kraft reduced-fat Cheddar cheese
> 2 tablespoons Hormel Bacon Bits
> 2 cups hot cooked spaghetti, rinsed and drained

In a large skillet sprayed with butter-flavored cooking spray, sauté chicken, onion, and green pepper for 5 minutes. Stir in chicken soup, water, undrained mushrooms, and undrained pimiento. Add Cheddar cheese and bacon bits. Mix well to combine. Fold in spaghetti. Lower heat and simmer for 5 to 6 minutes or until mixture is heated through and cheese melts, stirring occasionally.

HINTS: 1. If you don't have leftovers, purchase a chunk of cooked chicken breast from your local deli.
2. Usually 1½ cups broken uncooked spaghetti cooks to about 2 cups.

Each serving equals:

HE: 3 Protein • 1 Bread • ¾ Vegetable • ½ Slider • 18 Optional Calories

---

304 Calories • 8 gm Fat • 28 gm Protein • 30 gm Carbohydrate • 706 mg Sodium • 162 mg Calcium • 2 gm Fiber

---

DIABETIC EXCHANGES: 3 Meat • 1½ Starch/Carbohydrate • ½ Vegetable

Chicken Skillet Pie

Chicken and biscuits is an old-fashioned tradition, especially across the South of our nation. This easy "potpie" takes less time to prepare than the frozen kind—and tastes far, far better.   ☻   Serves 4

¾ cup sliced celery
¼ cup chopped onion
1 (10¾-ounce) can Healthy Request Cream of Chicken Soup
¼ cup fat-free milk
1 (8-ounce) can sliced carrots, rinsed and drained
1½ cups (8 ounces) diced cooked chicken breast
¾ cup Bisquick Reduced Fat Baking Mix
¼ cup water
1 teaspoon dried parsley flakes

In a large skillet sprayed with butter-flavored cooking spray, sauté celery and onion for 10 minutes. Stir in chicken soup and milk. Add carrots and chicken. Mix well to combine. Lower heat and simmer for 5 minutes, stirring occasionally. In a medium bowl, combine baking mix, water, and parsley flakes. Spread mixture evenly over chicken mixture. Cover and continue cooking for 5 minutes or until biscuit crust is firm. Divide into 4 servings.

HINT: If you don't have leftovers, purchase a chunk of cooked chicken breast from your local deli.

Each serving equals:

HE: 2 Protein • 1 Bread • 1 Vegetable • ½ Slider • 5 Optional Calories

245 Calories • 5 gm Fat • 22 gm Protein • 28 gm Carbohydrate • 751 mg Sodium • 72 mg Calcium • 2 gm Fiber

DIABETIC EXCHANGES: 2 Meat • 1½ Starch/Carbohydrate • 1 Vegetable

Western Chicken Breasts

I've breaded chicken in a variety of ways, but I really like the crunch that cornflakes provide. Here, the spices take a classic coating and set off a few fireworks! If you don't believe me, just ask my son James! ● Serves 4

> ¾ cup (¾ ounce) crushed cornflakes
> 1 teaspoon dried onion flakes
> 1 teaspoon dried parsley flakes
> ½ cup Kraft Fat Free French Dressing
> 1½ teaspoons chili seasoning
> 16 ounces skinned and boned uncooked chicken breast,
>   cut into 4 pieces

Preheat oven to 375 degrees. Spray a baking pan with butter-flavored cooking spray. In a medium bowl, combine cornflakes, onion flakes, and parsley flakes. In a sauce pan, combine French dressing and chili seasoning. Dip chicken pieces in dressing mixture, then roll in crumb mixture. Place chicken on prepared baking pan. Evenly spoon remaining sauce and crumbs over chicken pieces. Light spray tops with butter-flavored cooking spray. Bake for 25 to 30 minutes.

HINT: A self-seal sandwich bag works great for crushing cornflakes.

Each serving equals:

HE: 3 Protein • ¼ Bread • ½ Slider •
10 Optional Calories

---

187 Calories • 3 gm Fat • 23 gm Protein •
17 gm Carbohydrate • 418 mg Sodium •
15 mg Calcium • 1 gm Fiber

DIABETIC EXCHANGES: 3 Meat • ½ Starch/Carbohydrate

Baked Tex-Mex Chicken

This dish sizzles and dazzles with only a few simple ingredients, but they're more than enough to take plain old chicken breasts to an exciting new level! The contrast of the sour cream and salsa is wonderfully rich.　　◑　　Serves 4

⅓ cup Kraft fat-free mayonnaise
1 teaspoon chili seasoning
1 cup chunky salsa (mild, medium, or hot) ☆
16 ounces skinned and boned uncooked chicken breasts,
　　cut into 4 pieces
¼ cup Land O Lakes no-fat sour cream

Preheat oven to 350 degrees. Spray an 8-by-8-inch baking dish with butter-flavored cooking spray. In a medium bowl, combine mayonnaise, chili seasoning, and ¼ cup salsa. Evenly spread mixture on both sides of chicken pieces. Place chicken in prepared baking dish. Bake for 30 to 35 minutes. Place baking dish on a wire rack and let set for 5 minutes. Divide into 4 servings. When serving, top each piece with 3 tablespoons salsa and 1 tablespoon sour cream.

Each serving equals:

HE: 3 Protein • ½ Vegetable • ¼ Slider •
8 Optional Calories

149 Calories • 1 gm Fat • 27 gm Protein •
8 gm Carbohydrate • 485 mg Sodium •
108 mg Calcium • 0 gm Fiber

DIABETIC EXCHANGES: 3 Meat • ½ Vegetable •
½ Starch/Carbohydrate

Glazed Maple Orange Chicken

I know, I know, this one sounds a bit unusual, but trust me, these ingredients cook up into a spectacular combination that's worthy of serving to guests! It's sweet and savory, fruity and tangy, and all-around delectable. ☻   Serves 4

> *16 ounces skinned and boned uncooked chicken breast,*
> *   cut into 4 pieces*
> *¼ cup orange marmalade spreadable fruit*
> *¼ cup Log Cabin Sugar Free Maple Syrup*
> *1 tablespoon country style Dijon mustard*
> *2 teaspoons dried parsley flakes*

In a large skillet sprayed with butter-flavored cooking spray, brown chicken pieces for 4 to 6 minutes. In a small bowl, combine spreadable fruit and maple syrup. Stir in mustard and parsley flakes. Drizzle mixture evenly over chicken pieces. Lower heat and simmer for 6 to 8 minutes.

Each serving equals:

HE: 3 Protein • 1 Fruit • 10 Optional Calories

171 Calories • 3 gm Fat • 23 gm Protein •
13 mg Carbohydrate • 232 mg Sodium •
19 mg Calcium • 0 gm Fiber

DIABETIC EXCHANGES: 3 Meat • 1 Fruit

Honey Mustard
Chicken–Potato Bake

Sometimes I buy ready-cooked chicken, and other times I cook up chicken breasts to use in several meals. This fragrant casserole dish has very few ingredients but an abundance of savory goodness.

● Serves 4

> 3 cups (10 ounces) shredded loose-packed frozen potatoes
> 1 cup chopped onion
> 16 ounces skinned and boned uncooked chicken breast,
>   cut into 4 pieces
> ½ cup Kraft Fat Free Honey Mustard Dressing

Preheat oven to 400 degrees. Spray an 8-by-8-inch baking dish with butter-flavored cooking spray. Layer potatoes and onion in prepared baking dish. Evenly arrange chicken pieces over top. Drizzle 2 tablespoons Honey Mustard dressing over each piece of chicken. Cover and bake for 30 minutes. Uncover and continue baking for 15 to 20 minutes. Place baking dish on a wire rack and let set for 5 minutes. Divide into 4 servings.

HINT: Mr. Dell's frozen shredded potatoes are a good choice or raw shredded potatoes, rinsed and patted dry, may be used in place of frozen potatoes.

Each serving equals:

HE: 3 Protein • ½ Bread • ½ Vegetable • ½ Slider • 10 Optional Calories

236 Calories • 4 gm Fat • 26 gm Protein • 24 gm Carbohydrate • 415 mg Sodium • 21 mg Calcium • 3 gm Fiber

DIABETIC EXCHANGES: 3 Meat • 1 Starch/Carbohydrate • ½ Vegetable

Scalloped Carrots and Chicken

I usually use packaged bread cubes in this recipe, but if you find yourself with leftover crusty bread, you can cut up your own bits and pieces to stir in. This is a perfect pantry pride of a dish, with convenient canned chicken as its centerpiece.   ☻   Serves 4

½ cup chopped onion
1 (16-ounce) can sliced carrots, rinsed and drained
¾ cup (3 ounces) shredded Kraft reduced-fat Cheddar cheese
2 cups (3 ounces) unseasoned dry bread cubes
1 (5-ounce) can Hormel 97% Fat Free Breast of Chicken, packed in
    water, drained and flaked
1 (10¾-ounce) can Healthy Request Cream of Celery Soup
1 cup fat-free milk
1 teaspoon dried parsley flakes
½ teaspoon poultry seasoning

Preheat oven to 350 degrees. Spray an 8-by-8-inch baking dish with butter-flavored cooking spray. In a large skillet sprayed with butter-flavored cooking spray, sauté onion for 5 minutes or until tender. In a large bowl, combine onion, carrots, Cheddar cheese, bread cubes, and chicken. Add celery soup, milk, parsley flakes, and poultry seasoning. Mix well to combine. Spread mixture into prepared baking dish. Bake for 30 minutes. Place baking dish on a wire rack and let set for 5 minutes. Divide into 4 servings.

Each serving equals:

HE: 2¼ Protein • 1¼ Vegetable • 1 Bread •
¼ Fat-Free Milk • ½ Slider • 1 Optional Calorie

229 Calories • 9 gm Fat • 17 gm Protein •
20 gm Carbohydrate • 835 mg Sodium •
301 mg Calcium • 2 gm Fiber

DIABETIC EXCHANGES: 2 Meat • 1 Vegetable •
1 Starch/Carbohydrate

Layered Broccoli-Chicken Casserole

There's something special about layered dishes, perhaps because they seem like main dish "parfaits"! This recipe combines some basic ingredients in a way that is fresh and fun to make and to eat.

◐ Serves 6

> 1 cup (3 ounces) uncooked Minute Rice
> 1 cup chopped onion
> 1 (16-ounce) package frozen chopped broccoli
> 1 (5-ounce) can Hormel 97% Fat Free Breast of Chicken, packed in water, drained and flaked
> ¾ cup (3 ounces) shredded Kraft reduced-fat Cheddar cheese
> 1 (10¾-ounce) can Healthy Request Cream of Chicken Soup
> ½ cup fat-free milk

Preheat oven to 350 degrees. Spray a 9-by-9-inch cake pan with butter-flavored cooking spray. Spread uncooked instant rice in bottom of prepared cake pan. Sprinkle onion over rice. Layer frozen broccoli, chicken, and Cheddar cheese over onion. In a small bowl, combine chicken soup and milk. Evenly pour mixture over top. Cover and bake for 30 minutes. Uncover and continue baking for 15 minutes. Place cake pan on a wire rack and let set for 5 minutes. Divide into 6 servings.

Each serving equals:

HE: 1½ Protein • 1¼ Vegetable • ½ Bread •
¼ Slider • 17 Optional Calories

169 Calories • 5 gm Fat • 13 gm Protein •
18 gm Carbohydrate • 470 mg Sodium •
199 mg Calcium • 3 gm Fiber

DIABETIC EXCHANGES: 1½ Meat • 1 Vegetable • 1 Starch

Chicken Patties with Mushroom Sauce

I've often used canned chicken in salads, but I figured it would also make scrumptious patties not unlike crab cakes. The rich and creamy sauce is downright luxurious, and the mushrooms add something extra special to the mix.   ☻   Serves 4

> 2 (5-ounce) cans Swanson White Chicken, packed in water, drained and flaked
> 14 small fat-free saltine crackers, made into fine crumbs
> 2 teaspoons dried onion flakes
> 1/2 cup finely chopped celery
> 1/2 cup fat-free milk ☆
> 1 (10 3/4-ounce) can Healthy Request Cream of Chicken Soup
> 1 (2.5-ounce) jar sliced mushrooms, drained
> 1/8 teaspoon black pepper
> 1 teaspoon dried parsley flakes

Preheat oven to 350 degrees. Spray an 8-by-8-inch baking dish with butter-flavored cooking spray. In a large bowl, combine chicken, cracker crumbs, onion flakes, celery, and 1/4 cup milk. Mix well using hands. Using a 1/3 cup measuring cup as a guide, form into 4 patties. Place patties in prepared baking dish. In a small bowl, combine chicken soup, remaining 1/4 cup milk, mushrooms, black pepper, and parsley flakes. Evenly spoon sauce mixture over patties. Bake for 45 minutes. When serving, spoon sauce mixture evenly over top of patties.

HINT: A self-seal sandwich bag works great for crushing crackers.

Each serving equals:

HE: 2 1/2 Protein • 1/2 Bread • 1/2 Vegetable • 1/2 Slider • 6 Optional Calories

184 Calories • 4 gm Fat • 18 gm Protein • 19 gm Carbohydrate • 706 mg Sodium • 46 mg Calcium • 2 gm Fiber

DIABETIC EXCHANGES: 2 1/2 Meat • 1 Starch • 1/2 Vegetable

Creamy Turkey and Noodles

Sometimes it can get chilly without warning when you're traveling from town to town, and all you want for supper is something cozy, warm, and filling. This is a dish to fit the bill on brisk fall nights . . . or anytime at all. ○ Serves 4 (1 cup)

1 cup finely chopped celery
½ cup chopped onion
1 (10¾-ounce) can Healthy Request Cream of Chicken Soup
¼ cup fat-free milk
⅓ cup Land O Lakes no-fat sour cream
1 teaspoon dried parsley flakes
1 (2-ounce) jar chopped pimiento, undrained
⅛ teaspoon black pepper
1½ cups (8 ounces) diced cooked turkey breast
2 cups cooked noodles, rinsed and drained

In a large skillet sprayed with butter-flavored cooking spray, sauté celery and onion for 10 minutes. Stir in chicken soup, milk, sour cream, parsley flakes, undrained pimiento, and black pepper. Add turkey and noodles. Mix well to combine. Lower heat and simmer for 5 minutes, stirring occasionally.

HINTS: 1. If you don't have leftovers, purchase a chunk of cooked turkey breast from your local deli.
2. Usually 1¾ cups uncooked noodles cooks to about 2 cups.

Each serving equals:

HE: 2 Protein • 1 Bread • ¾ Vegetable • ¾ Slider •
5 Optional Calories

260 Calories • 4 gm Fat • 24 gm Protein •
32 gm Carbohydrate • 393 mg Sodium •
79 mg Calcium • 2 gm Fiber

DIABETIC EXCHANGES: 2 Meat •
1½ Starch/Carbohydrate • ½ Vegetable

Turkey Stovetop Dinner

I almost named this dish after my grandson's kaleidoscope—it's so colorful and full of flavors! What it is even more is a fast and festive way to serve leftover turkey, just perfect for those weeks between Thanksgiving and Christmas when you're almost too busy to cook.

○ Serves 6 (1 cup)

> 2 full cups (12 ounces) diced cooked turkey breast
> ½ cup chopped onion
> ½ cup chunky salsa (mild, medium, or hot)
> 1 (16-ounce) can tomatoes, chopped and undrained
> 1 (2-ounce) jar chopped pimiento, undrained
> ¾ cup water
> 1 tablespoon Splenda Granular
> 1 teaspoon dried parsley flakes
> 1 cup frozen whole-kernel corn, thawed
> 1⅓ cups (4 ounces) uncooked Minute Rice

In a large skillet sprayed with butter-flavored cooking spray, sauté turkey and onion for 5 minutes. Add salsa, undrained tomatoes, undrained pimiento, water, Splenda, and parsley flakes. Mix well to combine. Bring mixture to a boil. Stir in corn and uncooked instant rice. Lower heat, cover, and simmer for 10 to 12 minutes or until rice is tender and most of liquid is absorbed, stirring occasionally.

HINTS: 1. If you don't have leftovers, purchase a chunk of cooked turkey breast from your local deli.
2. Thaw corn by placing in a colander and rinsing under hot water for 1 minute.

Each serving equals:

HE: 2 Protein • 1 Bread • 1 Vegetable •
1 Optional Calorie

---

199 Calories • 3 gm Fat • 20 gm Protein •
23 gm Carbohydrate • 293 mg Sodium •
33 mg Calcium • 2 gm Fiber

DIABETIC EXCHANGES: 2 Meat • 1 Starch • 1 Vegetable

Rice Olé

You could almost write a poem about this dish, something along the lines of "So nice, so nice, mix up cheese and meat and rice, and you'll want to eat it twice!" I guess I was inspired by a taste!

○ Serves 4 (1 cup)

> 8 ounces extra-lean ground sirloin beef or turkey breast
> ½ cup chopped onion
> 1 (15-ounce) can Hunt's Tomato Sauce
> ½ cup water
> 1 teaspoon chili seasoning
> 1 tablespoon Splenda Granular
> ¾ cup (3 ounces) shredded Kraft reduced-fat Cheddar cheese
> 1⅓ cups (4 ounces) uncooked Minute Rice

In a large skillet sprayed with olive oil–flavored cooking spray, brown meat and onion. Stir in tomato sauce, water, chili seasoning, Splenda, and Cheddar cheese. Continue cooking until cheese melts and mixture starts to boil, stirring often. Add uncooked instant rice. Mix well to combine. Lower heat, cover, and simmer for 6 to 8 minutes or until rice is tender, stirring occasionally.

Each serving equals:

HE: 2½ Protein • 2 Vegetable • 1 Bread •
2 Optional Calories

232 Calories • 8 gm Fat • 18 gm Protein •
22 gm Carbohydrate • 882 mg Sodium •
163 mg Calcium • 2 gm Fiber

DIABETIC EXCHANGES: 2 Meat • 2 Vegetable • 1 Starch

South of the Border
Macaroni and Cheese

Classic mac and cheese omits any mention of meat, but if you've got cheeseburger fans in the family (and who doesn't!), you'll love this version that blends some salsa and meat into the well-loved standard. Go as hot and spicy as you dare—but please remember the "wimpy" family members (like me!) before you pour on the heat.

○ Serves 4 (1 cup)

> 8 ounces extra-lean ground sirloin beef or turkey breast
> 1 cup chunky salsa (mild, medium, or hot)
> ¾ cup water
> 1⅓ cups (3 ounces) uncooked elbow macaroni
> ¾ cup (3 ounces) shredded Kraft reduced-fat Cheddar cheese
> ¼ cup Land O Lakes no-fat sour cream
> 1 teaspoon dried parsley flakes

In a large skillet sprayed with olive oil–flavored cooking spray, brown meat. Stir in salsa and water. Bring mixture to a boil. Add uncooked macaroni. Mix well to combine. Lower heat, cover, and simmer for 10 minutes or until macaroni is tender, stirring occasionally. Stir in Cheddar cheese, sour cream, and parsley flakes. Continue cooking until cheese is melted and mixture is heated through, stirring occasionally.

Each serving equals:

HE: 2½ Protein • 1 Bread • ½ Vegetable •
15 Optional Calories

---

242 Calories • 6 gm Fat • 22 gm Protein •
25 gm Carbohydrate • 671 mg Sodium •
165 mg Calcium • 3 gm Fiber

DIABETIC EXCHANGES: 2½ Meat • 1 Starch •
½ Vegetable

Cliff's Special Skillet

I don't know what we did before the big warehouse stores allowed us to buy case lots of canned green beans, but we're never without at least a dozen cans of Cliff's favorite vegetable! This skillet supper surrounds those green beauties with the kind of meat-and-potatoes flavor a man's just gotta love. ☺ Serves 4 (1 cup)

> 8 ounces extra-lean ground sirloin beef or turkey breast
> ½ cup finely chopped onion
> 1 (10¾-ounce) can Healthy Request Tomato Soup
> 2 teaspoons dried parsley flakes
> ⅛ teaspoon black pepper
> 1 (16-ounce) can cut green beans, rinsed and drained
> 2 full cups (12 ounces) diced cooked potatoes

In a large skillet sprayed with butter-flavored cooking spray, brown meat and onion. Stir in tomato soup, parsley flakes, and black pepper. Add green beans and potatoes. Mix well to combine. Lower heat and simmer for 6 to 8 minutes or until mixture is heated through, stirring occasionally.

Each serving equals:

HE: 1½ Protein • 1¼ Vegetable • ¾ Bread •
½ Slider • 5 Optional Calories

---

220 Calories • 4 gm Fat • 14 gm Protein •
32 gm Carbohydrate • 609 mg Sodium •
30 mg Calcium • 4 gm Fiber

DIABETIC EXCHANGES: 1½ Meat •
1½ Starch/Carbohydrate • 1 Vegetable

Country Cousin Skillet

Whether you're a city girl or a woman who can't truly be happy anywhere but on a farm, you're bound to love this meat-and-veggie dish that celebrates the homey goodness of corn.

○ Serves 4 (1 cup)

8 ounces extra-lean ground sirloin beef or turkey breast
½ cup chopped onion
½ cup chopped green bell pepper
1 (16-ounce) can tomatoes, coarsely chopped and undrained
1 teaspoon dried parsley flakes
⅛ teaspoon black pepper
2 cups frozen whole-kernel corn, thawed

In a large skillet sprayed with butter-flavored cooking spray, brown meat, onion, and green pepper. Stir in undrained tomatoes, parsley flakes, and black pepper. Add corn. Mix well to combine. Lower heat and simmer for 5 minutes or until mixture is heated through, stirring occasionally.

HINT: Thaw corn by placing in a colander and rinsing under hot water for 1 minute.

Each serving equals:

HE: 1½ Protein • 1½ Vegetable • 1 Bread

188 Calories • 4 gm Fat • 15 gm Protein •
23 gm Carbohydrate • 256 mg Sodium • 30 mg Calcium

DIABETIC EXCHANGES: 1½ Meat • 1½ Vegetable •
1 Starch

Unstuffed Cabbage Skillet

I've dined on homemade stuffed cabbage in kitchens across the United States, but some days you just don't have the means or the time to prepare this beloved supper the old-fashioned way. Try this skillet version for a speedy supper sometime—and see if you don't see smiles all around the table!   ☾   Serves 4 (1 cup)

8 ounces extra-lean ground sirloin beef or turkey breast
½ cup chopped onion
1 (10¾-ounce) can Healthy Request Tomato Soup
1⅓ cups water
1 teaspoon Worcestershire sauce
1 teaspoon prepared yellow mustard
1 teaspoon dried parsley flakes
1⅓ cups (4 ounces) uncooked Minute Rice
2 cups shredded cabbage

In a large skillet sprayed with butter-flavored cooking spray, brown meat and onion. Stir in tomato soup, water, Worcestershire sauce, mustard, and parsley flakes. Bring mixture to a boil. Add rice and cabbage. Mix well to combine. Lower heat, cover, and simmer for 15 minutes or until rice and cabbage are tender, stirring occasionally.

Each serving equals:

HE: 1½ Protein • 1¾ Vegetable • 1 Bread •
½ Slider • 5 Optional Calories

233 Calories • 5 gm Fat • 15 gm Protein •
32 gm Carbohydrate • 355 mg Sodium •
36 mg Calcium • 3 gm Fiber

DIABETIC EXCHANGES: 1½ Meat •
1½ Starch/Carbohydrate • 1 Vegetable

Celery Stroganoff over English Muffins

Here's a recipe designed to serve six, but if you're just two for dinner tonight, you could easily reheat the creamy mixture in the microwave tomorrow and enjoy it again. My daughter-in-law Pam loves creamy dishes like this one, at home or on the road.   ☻   Serves 6

16 ounces extra-lean ground sirloin beef or turkey breast
1 cup finely chopped celery
½ cup finely chopped onion
1 (10¾-ounce) can Healthy Request Cream of Celery Soup
¼ cup Land O Lakes no-fat sour cream
1 teaspoon dried parsley flakes
⅛ teaspoon black pepper
3 English muffins, split and toasted

In a large skillet sprayed with butter-flavored cooking spray, brown meat, celery, and onion. Stir in celery soup, sour cream, parsley flakes, and black pepper. Lower heat and simmer for 10 minutes, stirring occasionally. For each serving, place an English muffin half on a plate and spoon about ½ cup sauce over top.

Each serving equals:

HE: 2 Protein • 1 Bread • ½ Vegetable • ¼ Slider •
18 Optional Calories

197 Calories • 5 gm Fat • 18 gm Protein •
20 gm Carbohydrate • 411 mg Sodium •
118 mg Calcium • 2 gm Fiber

DIABETIC EXCHANGES: 2 Meat • 1 Starch • ½ Vegetable

Grandma's
Spaghetti Skillet Stew

What a fun and flavorful one-pot meal that is good enough to win Grandma's approval! Brimming with a little bit of this and that, it's as hearty as it is thrifty, so it's just about perfect for any family, anytime.

○ Serves 4 (1 cup)

> 2 cups shredded cabbage
> ½ cup chopped onion
> 1 cup shredded carrots
> 1 (14½-ounce) can Swanson Beef Broth
> ¼ cup water
> 1 teaspoon dried parsley flakes
> ⅛ teaspoon black pepper
> 1½ cups (8 ounces) diced cooked lean roast beef
> 1½ cups (3 ounces) broken uncooked spaghetti

In a large skillet sprayed with butter-flavored cooking spray, sauté cabbage, onion, and carrots for 5 minutes. Add beef broth, water, parsley flakes, black pepper, and roast beef. Mix well to combine. Stir in uncooked spaghetti. Lower heat, cover, and simmer for 15 minutes or until spaghetti and vegetables are tender, stirring occasionally.

Each serving equals:

HE: 2 Protein • 1¼ Vegetable • 1 Bread •
8 Optional Calories

226 Calories • 6 gm Fat • 21 gm Protein •
22 gm Carbohydrate • 407 mg Sodium •
35 mg Calcium • 2 gm Fiber

DIABETIC EXCHANGES: 2 Meat • 1 Vegetable • 1 Starch

Yankee Chili Skillet

One of the best-loved dishes in all of New England is Yankee bean soup, so that was part of my inspiration for this savory skillet supper. But it also makes good Yankee sense to use up bits of leftovers in this dish—some carrots, maybe some leftover macaroni, even half an onion looking lonely in the fridge!   ♥   Serves 4 (1¼ cups)

> 8 ounces extra-lean ground sirloin beef or turkey breast
> ½ cup chopped onion
> ½ cup chopped green bell pepper
> 1 cup shredded carrots
> 1 cup chopped celery
> 1 (10¾-ounce) can Healthy Request Tomato Soup
> 1 (14½-ounce) can Swanson Beef Broth
> 2 teaspoons chili seasoning
> 1 (8-ounce) can red kidney beans, rinsed and drained
> 1 cup (2¼ ounces) uncooked elbow macaroni

In a large skillet sprayed with butter-flavored cooking spray, brown meat, onion, green pepper, carrots, and celery for 10 minutes. Add tomato soup, beef broth, and chili seasoning. Mix well to combine. Bring mixture to a boil. Stir in kidney beans and uncooked macaroni. Lower heat and simmer for 10 to 12 minutes, or until macaroni is tender, stirring occasionally.

Each serving equals:

HE: 2¼ Protein • 1½ Vegetable • ¾ Bread •
½ Slider • 14 Optional Calories

244 Calories • 4 gm Fat • 18 gm Protein •
34 gm Carbohydrate • 859 mg Sodium •
48 mg Calcium • 8 gm Fiber

DIABETIC EXCHANGES: 1½ Meat • 1½ Vegetable •
1½ Starch/Carbohydrate

Rio Grande Spaghetti Skillet

They say that everything is bigger in Texas, and I've eaten enough Texas-style meals to agree with that saying. This one-pot supper delivers a ton of taste with very little fuss—and the spirit of Texas cooking is alive in every mouthful!   ☻   Serves 4 (1 cup)

> 8 ounces extra-lean ground sirloin beef or turkey breast
> ½ cup chopped onion
> ½ cup chopped green bell pepper
> 2 cups reduced-sodium tomato juice
> ½ cup water
> 1 tablespoon Splenda
> 1½ teaspoons taco seasoning
> 1¾ cups (3 ounces) broken uncooked spaghetti
> ¼ cup (1 ounce) sliced ripe olives
> ¼ cup Land O Lakes no-fat sour cream

In a large skillet sprayed with olive oil–flavored cooking spray, brown meat, onion, and green pepper. Add tomato juice, water, Splenda, and taco seasoning. Mix well to combine. Bring mixture to a boil. Stir in uncooked spaghetti and olives. Lower heat, cover, and simmer for 20 to 24 minutes or until spaghetti is tender, stirring occasionally. When serving, top each serving with 1 tablespoon sour cream.

Each serving equals:

HE: 1½ Protein • 1½ Vegetable • 1 Bread • ¼ Fat •
16 Optional Calories

217 Calories • 5 gm Fat • 18 gm Protein •
25 gm Carbohydrate • 202 mg Sodium •
63 mg Calcium • 2 gm Fiber

DIABETIC EXCHANGES: 1½ Meat • 1½ Vegetable •
1 Starch

Salisbury Spaghetti Skillet

We're all trying to eat healthier these days, which often means less meat and more grains (like pasta). But if your family longs for truly hearty meals, here's a way to serve up loads of meaty flavor without the calories and fat. ☻ Serves 4 (1 cup)

8 ounces extra-lean ground sirloin beef or turkey breast
½ cup chopped onion
1 (12-ounce) jar Heinz Fat Free Beef Gravy
1¼ cups water
¼ cup reduced-sodium ketchup
2 teaspoons dried parsley flakes
1 (2.5-ounce) jar sliced mushrooms, undrained
⅛ teaspoon black pepper
1¾ cups (3 ounces) broken uncooked spaghetti

In a large skillet sprayed with butter-flavored cooking spray, brown meat and onion. Add beef gravy, water, and ketchup. Mix well to combine. Bring mixture to a boil. Stir in parsley flakes, undrained mushrooms, black pepper, and uncooked spaghetti. Lower heat, cover, and simmer for 18 to 20 minutes or until spaghetti is tender, stirring occasionally.

Each serving equals:

HE: 1½ Protein • 1 Bread • ½ Vegetable • ½ Slider • 12 Optional Calories

---

200 Calories • 4 gm Fat • 16 gm Protein • 25 gm Carbohydrate • 609 mg Sodium • 15 mg Calcium • 2 gm Fiber

---

DIABETIC EXCHANGES: 1½ Meat • 1½ Starch/Carbohydrate • ½ Vegetable

Italian Twist Skillet

Imagine you're driving between Rome and Florence instead of across the Midwestern plains. To make the daydream just about perfect, why not serve this *bellissima* pasta dish that will convince your mouth you're in Italy for supper!   ● Serves 4 (1 cup)

> 8 ounces extra-lean ground sirloin beef or turkey breast
> 1 (14½-ounce) can Swanson Beef Broth
> ⅓ cup water
> 2 teaspoons Worcestershire sauce
> 1 teaspoon Italian seasoning
> 1 (8-ounce) can stewed tomatoes, coarsely chopped and undrained
> 1½ cups (3 ounces) uncooked rotini pasta
> ¼ cup (¾ ounce) Kraft Reduced Fat Parmesan Style Grated
>   Topping

In a large skillet sprayed with olive oil–flavored cooking spray, brown meat. Stir in beef broth, water, Worcestershire sauce, Italian seasoning, and undrained stewed tomatoes. Bring mixture to a boil. Add uncooked rotini pasta. Mix well to combine. Lower heat, cover, and simmer for 10 minutes. Uncover and continue cooking for 5 minutes or until pasta is tender and most of liquid is absorbed, stirring occasionally. Add Parmesan cheese. Mix gently to combine. Serve at once.

Each serving equals:

HE: 1¾ Protein • 1 Bread • ½ Vegetable •
5 Optional Calories

144 Calories • 4 gm Fat • 14 gm Protein •
13 gm Carbohydrate • 556 mg Sodium •
57 mg Calcium • 1 gm Fiber

DIABETIC EXCHANGES: 2 Meat • 1 Starch/Carbohydrate •
½ Vegetable

Pepper Steak Gravy over Garlic Potatoes

Green peppers are usually the thriftiest peppers you can buy—almost always less expensive than red or yellow. They are the perfect partner to the rich beef flavor this recipe provides, and a fine contrast to creamy mashed potatoes, too! ☻ Serves 4

> 8 ounces extra-lean ground sirloin beef or turkey breast
> 1½ cups chopped green bell pepper
> ½ cup chopped onion
> 1 (2-ounce) jar chopped pimiento, drained
> 1 (12-ounce) can Heinz Fat Free Beef Gravy
> 1⅔ cups hot water
> 1⅓ cups instant potato flakes
> ¼ teaspoon dried minced garlic
> ¼ cup Land O Lakes no-fat sour cream

In a large skillet sprayed with butter-flavored cooking spray, brown meat, green pepper, and onion. Stir in pimiento and beef gravy. Lower heat and simmer while preparing potatoes, stirring occasionally. In a medium saucepan, bring water to a boil. Remove from heat and add potato flakes and garlic. Mix gently to combine, using a fork. Stir in sour cream. For each serving, place about ½ cup potatoes on a plate and spoon a full ½ cup meat gravy over top.

Each serving equals:

HE: 1½ Protein • 1 Bread • 1 Vegetable • ½ Slider •
12 Optional Calories

---

187 Calories • 3 gm Fat • 15 gm Protein •
25 gm Carbohydrate • 537 mg Sodium •
38 mg Calcium • 3 gm Fiber

DIABETIC EXCHANGES: 1½ Meat •
1½ Starch/Carbohydrate • ½ Vegetable

Layered Cabbage Meat Bake

Sometimes I get an idea for a recipe that I'm not at all certain will work as I envision it, but I'm determined to try it—and keep trying until I get it right! This dish looked a bit unusual before I slipped it into the oven, but if you've got time for a little magic, you'll be very pleased with the results. ○ Serves 6

16 ounces extra-lean ground sirloin beef or turkey breast
1½ cups chopped onion
6 cups shredded cabbage ☆
1 (10¾-ounce) can Healthy Request Tomato Soup
1 teaspoon chili seasoning
⅛ teaspoon black pepper

Preheat oven to 350 degrees. In a large skillet sprayed with butter-flavored cooking spray, brown meat and onion. Spread 3 cups cabbage in deep dish 9-inch pie plate. Evenly spoon meat mixture over cabbage. Cover with remaining 3 cups cabbage. In a small bowl, combine tomato soup, chili seasoning, and black pepper. Evenly spoon soup mixture over top. Cover and bake for 1 hour. Place baking dish on a wire rack and let set for 5 minutes. Divide into 6 servings.

Each serving equals:

HE: 2 Protein • 1½ Vegetable • ¼ Slider • 10 Optional Calories

---

171 Calories • 7 gm Fat • 15 gm Protein • 12 gm Carbohydrate • 238 mg Sodium • 44 mg Calcium • 2 gm Fiber

---

DIABETIC EXCHANGES: 2 Meat • 1½ Vegetable

Nacho Crescent Bake

When you're traveling with kids, it's good to have a few recipes designed to win their hearts and taste buds—and this dish deserves to be called "Fun Food!" Instead of pulling into a fast-food Mexican restaurant, give them these truly tasty nachos for supper.

○ Serves 6

> 8 ounces extra-lean ground sirloin beef or turkey breast
> ½ cup chopped onion
> 1 (10¾-ounce) can Healthy Request Tomato Soup ☆
> 1 teaspoon taco seasoning
> 1 (8-ounce) can Pillsbury Reduced Fat Crescent Rolls
> ¾ cup (3 ounces) shredded Kraft reduced-fat Cheddar cheese
> ¾ cup chunky salsa (mild, medium, or hot)

Preheat oven to 375 degrees. In a large skillet sprayed with butter-flavored cooking spray, brown meat and onion. Stir in ½ cup tomato soup and taco seasoning. Lower heat and simmer for 5 minutes, stirring occasionally. Meanwhile, on a large baking sheet sprayed with butter-flavored cooking spray, unroll crescent rolls. Evenly spoon meat mixture over rolls. Roll up like a jelly roll starting with long side. Seal edge well. Place sealed edge down. Curve into a large crescent shape. Gently make several slashes in top. Evenly sprinkle Cheddar cheese over top. Bake for 12 to 16 minutes or until crust is golden brown. Place baking sheet on a wire rack and let set for 5 minutes. Meanwhile, in a small saucepan, combine remaining tomato soup and salsa. Cook over medium heat for 3 to 4 minutes or until mixture is heated through. Cut crescent into 6 pieces. For each serving, place 1 piece on a plate and spoon a full 3 tablespoons sauce mixture over top.

Each serving equals:

> HE: 1½ Protein • 1¼ Bread • ¼ Vegetable •
> ½ Slider • 5 Optional Calories
>
> ---
>
> 196 Calories • 9 gm Fat • 15 gm Protein •
> 26 gm Carbohydrate • 705 mg Sodium •
> 100 mg Calcium • 1 gm Fiber
>
> ---
>
> DIABETIC EXCHANGES: 1½ Meat • 1½ Starch • ½ Fat

Tomato Basil Meat Loaf

It's truly amazing what a wallop of great taste just a bit of dried spice can bring to a classic meat loaf recipe. I like to crumble the basil into the dish to release every last bit of flavor it has hidden in each leaf.

● Serves 6

> 16 ounces extra-lean ground sirloin beef or turkey breast
> ½ cup + 1 tablespoon dried fine bread crumbs
> 2 teaspoons dried basil leaves ☆
> ¾ cup finely chopped onion
> 1 (10¾-ounce) can Healthy Request Tomato Soup ☆

Preheat oven to 350 degrees. Spray a 9-by-5-inch loaf pan with olive oil–flavored cooking spray. In a large bowl, combine meat, bread crumbs, 1 teaspoon basil, onion, and ⅓ cup tomato soup. Mix well to combine. Pat mixture into prepared loaf pan. Bake for 40 minutes. Stir remaining 1 teaspoon basil into remaining tomato soup. Evenly spoon soup mixture over partially baked meat loaf. Continue baking for 15 minutes. Place loaf pan on a wire rack and let set for 5 minutes. Cut into 6 servings.

Each serving equals:

> HE: 2 Protein • ½ Bread • ¼ Vegetable • ¼ Slider •
> 10 Optional Calories
>
> ---
>
> 160 Calories • 4 gm Fat • 16 gm Protein •
> 15 gm Carbohydrate • 293 mg Sodium •
> 36 mg Calcium • 1 gm Fiber
>
> ---
>
> DIABETIC EXCHANGES: 2 Meat • 1 Starch/Carbohydrate

Home Style Meat Loaf with Cheese Sauce

I've stirred up dozens of meat loaf recipes over the years, and each one has been a favorite of someone in my family. Well, when I tested this one at a big gathering of the clan not long ago, it was voted a winner by just about everyone at the table! ☻ Serves 6

16 ounces extra-lean ground sirloin beef or turkey breast
½ cup + 1 tablespoon dried fine bread crumbs
2 teaspoons dried parsley flakes ☆
2 teaspoons dried onion flakes ☆
1 (12-fluid-ounce) can Carnation Evaporated Fat Free Milk ☆
1 (10¾-ounce) can Healthy Request Cream of Mushroom Soup
¾ cup (3 ounces) shredded Kraft reduced-fat Cheddar cheese

Preheat oven to 350 degrees. Spray a 9-by-5-inch loaf pan with butter-flavored cooking spray. In a large bowl, combine meat, bread crumbs, 1 teaspoon parsley flakes, 1 teaspoon onion flakes, and ½ cup evaporated milk. Mix well to combine. Pat mixture into prepared loaf pan. Bake for 50 to 55 minutes. Place loaf pan on a wire rack and let set for 5 minutes. Meanwhile, in a medium saucepan, combine mushroom soup, remaining 1 cup evaporated milk, remaining 1 teaspoon parsley flakes, and remaining 1 teaspoon onion flakes. Stir in Cheddar cheese. Cook over medium heat for 5 minutes or until cheese melts, stirring often. Cut meat loaf into 6 servings. For each serving, place 1 piece of meatloaf on a plate and spoon about ⅓ cup cheese sauce over top.

Each serving equals:

HE: 2½ Protein • ½ Fat-Free Milk • ½ Bread •
¼ Slider • 18 Optional Calories

239 Calories • 7 gm Fat • 24 gm Protein •
20 gm Carbohydrate • 530 mg Sodium •
320 mg Calcium • 0 gm Fiber

DIABETIC EXCHANGES: 2½ Meat •
1 Starch/Carbohydrate • ½ Fat-Free Milk

Country Stroganoff with Rice

Here's a terrific way to use up leftover roast beef, or to make something great for dinner when the only place you can shop is a deli! This dish is best with fresh mushrooms, but in a pinch you can substitute the canned kind.   ☺   Serves 4

1½ cups (8 ounces) diced cooked lean roast beef
½ cup chopped onion
1½ cups sliced fresh mushrooms
1 (10¾-ounce) can Healthy Request Cream of Mushroom Soup
¼ cup water
2 tablespoons country style Dijon mustard
1 teaspoon dried parsley flakes
¼ cup Land O Lakes no-fat sour cream
2 cups hot cooked rice

In a large skillet sprayed with butter-flavored cooking spray, sauté roast beef and onion for 3 minutes. Stir in mushrooms. Add mushroom soup, water, mustard, parsley flakes, and sour cream. Mix gently to combine. Lower heat and simmer for 5 to 6 minutes or until mixture is heated through, stirring occasionally. For each serving, place ½ cup rice on a plate and spoon about ¾ cup meat mixture over top.

HINT: Usually 1⅓ cups uncooked instant rice cooks to about 2 cups.

Each serving equals:

HE: 2 Protein • 1 Bread • 1 Vegetable • ½ Slider • 16 Optional Calories

259 Calories • 7 gm Fat • 20 gm Protein • 29 gm Carbohydrate • 507 mg Sodium • 97 mg Calcium • 1 gm Fiber

DIABETIC EXCHANGES: 2 Meat • 1½ Starch • ½ Vegetable

One Dish Stroganoff with Noodles

When I first started testing fat-free sour cream, I was concerned about how it would cook—whether or not it would get watery or separate. The good news is that you can make blissfully creamy dishes with these exciting products, and you don't have to worry for an instant! ☻ Serves 4 (1 cup)

8 ounces lean round steak, cut into 24 pieces
½ cup chopped onion
1 (14½-ounce) can Swanson Beef Broth
1 (10¾-ounce) can Healthy Request Cream of Mushroom Soup
1 (2.5-ounce) jar sliced mushrooms, drained
1¾ cups (3 ounces) uncooked noodles
¼ cup Land O Lakes no-fat sour cream

In a large skillet sprayed with butter-flavored cooking spray, brown meat and onion for 8 to 10 minutes. Stir in beef broth and mushroom soup. Bring mixture to a boil. Add mushrooms and uncooked noodles. Mix well to combine. Lower heat and simmer for 10 minutes or until noodles are tender, stirring occasionally. Stir in sour cream. Continue simmering for 2 to 3 minutes or until mixture is heated through, stirring occasionally.

Each serving equals:

HE: 1½ Protein • 1 Bread • ½ Vegetable • ½ Slider • 5 Optional Calories

250 Calories • 6 gm Fat • 25 gm Protein • 24 gm Carbohydrate • 708 mg Sodium • 96 mg Calcium • 1 gm Fiber

DIABETIC EXCHANGES: 1½ Meat • 1½ Starch • ½ Vegetable

Stuffed Beef Rolls

This looks fancy enough for company, but it's a smart and simple way to make steaks a little bit special on any night at all! Make sure you place the rolled-up steaks "seam-side" down so they don't open up.

❍ Serves 4

3 tablespoons dried fine bread crumbs
1 teaspoon dried onion flakes
¼ cup hot water
4 (4 ounce) lean minute or cube steaks
1 (15-ounce) can Hunt's Tomato Sauce
1 teaspoon dried parsley flakes
⅛ teaspoon black pepper
1 tablespoon Splenda Granular

In a small bowl, combine bread crumbs, onion flakes, and water. Evenly spoon a full tablespoon stuffing mixture over center of each steak. Roll steaks over stuffing mixture and secure with a toothpick. Place rolled steaks in a large skillet sprayed with butter-flavored cooking spray. Brown for 2 to 3 minutes on each side. In a small bowl, combine tomato sauce, parsley flakes, black pepper, and Splenda. Spoon mixture evenly over steaks. Lower heat, cover, and simmer for 30 minutes, or until meat is tender. When serving, evenly spoon sauce mixture over beef rolls.

Each serving equals:

HE: 3 Protein • 1¾ Vegetable • ¼ Bread •
1 Optional Calorie

234 Calories • 6 gm Fat • 28 gm Protein •
17 gm Carbohydrate • 831 mg Sodium •
21 mg Calcium • 2 gm Fiber

DIABETIC EXCHANGES: 3 Meat • 1½ Vegetable

Skillet Beef and Vegetables

As long as you keep it lean, you can happily keep steak on the menu, which is a real comfort to most of the men I know! Here's a way to be sure they're also getting their vegetables, but in a dish that is so downright delicious they'll gobble up every bite.

☻ Serves 4

8 ounces lean round steak, cut into 24 pieces
½ cup chopped onion
3 cups frozen broccoli, carrot, and cauliflower blend, thawed
1 (12-ounce) jar Heinz Fat Free Beef Gravy
1 teaspoon dried parsley flakes
⅛ teaspoon black pepper
2 cups hot cooked noodles, rinsed and drained

In a large skillet sprayed with butter-flavored cooking spray, sauté steak, onion, and vegetable blend for 10 minutes. Stir in beef gravy, parsley flakes, and black pepper. Lower heat and simmer for 10 minutes, stirring occasionally. For each serving, place ½ cup noodles on a plate and spoon about ¾ cup steak mixture over top.

HINTS: 1. Thaw vegetable blend by placing in a colander and rinsing under hot water for 1 minute.
2. Usually 1¾ cups uncooked noodles cooks to about 2 cups.

Each serving equals:

HE: 1¾ Vegetable • 1½ Protein • 1 Bread •
¼ Slider • 18 Optional Calories

285 Calories • 5 gm Fat • 28 gm Protein •
32 gm Carbohydrate • 565 mg Sodium •
58 mg Calcium • 4 gm Fiber

DIABETIC EXCHANGES: 2 Vegetable • 1½ Meat •
1½ Starch

Smothered Steak and Onions over Noodles

When I stock my freezer for a getaway, I look for great bargains on meat—and lean round steak is one of Cliff's favorites. Served with a tasty gravy and piles of noodles, it's a meal any man will love!

○ Serves 6

> 16 ounces lean round steak, cut into 36 pieces
> 2½ cups sliced onion
> 1 (12-ounce) jar Heinz Fat Free Beef Gravy
> 1 (10¾-ounce) can Healthy Request Cream of Mushroom Soup
> 1 (2.5-ounce) jar sliced mushrooms, undrained
> 2 teaspoons dried parsley flakes
> ⅛ teaspoon black pepper
> 3 cups hot cooked noodles, rinsed and drained

In a large skillet sprayed with butter-flavored cooking spray, sauté steak pieces and onion for 6 to 8 minutes. Stir in beef gravy and mushroom soup. Add undrained mushrooms, parsley flakes, and black pepper. Mix well to combine. Lower heat, cover, and simmer for 20 to 25 minutes, or until meat is tender. For each serving, place ½ cup noodles on a plate and spoon about ⅔ cup steak mixture over top.

HINT: Usually 2⅔ cups uncooked noodles cooks to about 3 cups.

Each serving equals:

> HE: 2 Protein • 1 Bread • 1 Vegetable • ½ Slider •
> 12 Optional Calories
>
> ---
> 269 Calories • 5 gm Fat • 24 gm Protein •
> 32 gm Carbohydrate • 643 mg Sodium •
> 70 mg Calcium • 2 gm Fiber
>
> ---
> DIABETIC EXCHANGES: 2 Meat •
> 1½ Starch/Carbohydrate • 1 Vegetable

Minute Steaks in Onion-Mushroom Gravy

My son Tom always loved these little steaks when he was growing up, and his wife Angie told me that he still does. Here's a fast and flavorful way to serve them soon!   ☻   Serves 4

4 (4-ounce) lean minute or cube steaks
1½ cups sliced onion
1 (2.5-ounce) jar sliced mushrooms, drained
1 (12-ounce) can Heinz Fat Free Beef Gravy
¼ cup Land O Lakes no-fat sour cream
1 teaspoon dried parsley flakes

In a large skillet sprayed with butter-flavored cooking spray, lightly brown meat for about 4 minutes on each side. Evenly sprinkle onion and mushrooms over top. In a medium bowl, combine beef gravy, sour cream, and parsley flakes. Spoon gravy mixture evenly over top. Lower heat, cover, and simmer for 30 minutes or until meat is tender. When serving, evenly spoon gravy mixture over meat.

Each serving equals:

HE: 3 Protein • 1 Vegetable • ½ Slider •
12 Optional Calories

217 Calories • 5 gm Fat • 30 gm Protein •
13 gm Carbohydrate • 604 mg Sodium •
40 mg Calcium • 1 gm Fiber

DIABETIC EXCHANGES: 3 Meat • 1 Vegetable •
½ Starch/Carbohydrate

Hot Dog Wraps

I invented this dish on a night when I was out of hot dog buns and Cliff and I were in the mood for hot dogs. (Remember what they say about necessity being the mother of invention?) This is the kind of dish children will love, too, because it's cheesy and oh-so-easy to eat! ☻   Serves 4

8 ounces Healthy Choice 97% fat-free frankfurters, diced
¾ cup (3 ounces) shredded Kraft reduced-fat Cheddar cheese
½ cup chunky salsa (mild, medium, or hot)
1 cup shredded lettuce
4 (6-inch) flour tortillas

In a large skillet sprayed with olive oil–flavored cooking spray, combine frankfurters, Cheddar cheese, and salsa. Cook over low heat until cheese melts, stirring often. For each wrap, place ¼ cup lettuce on a tortilla, spoon a full ⅓ cup frankfurter mixture over top, and roll up jelly-roll fashion. Serve at once.

Each serving equals:

HE: 2¼ Protein • 1 Bread • ½ Vegetable

211 Calories • 7 gm Fat • 15 gm Protein •
22 gm Carbohydrate • 956 mg Sodium •
198 mg Calcium • 0 gm Fiber

DIABETIC EXCHANGES: 2 Meat • 1 Starch •
½ Vegetable

Chuck Wagon Supper

Here's a fun family meal that takes so little time to stir up, you won't have to miss a moment of the splendid scenery rushing past! It's protein-rich, with its mix of beans and franks, but even more important, it's a tummy-pleasing solution to that age-old query, "What's for dinner, Mom?"   ❂   Serves 4 (1 cup)

½ cup chopped onion
8 ounces Healthy Choice 97% fat-free frankfurters, diced
1 (8-ounce) can Hunt's Tomato Sauce
2 tablespoons Hormel Bacon Bits
2 tablespoons Splenda Granular
1 tablespoon prepared yellow mustard
1 (16-ounce) can pinto beans, rinsed and drained
1 cup hot cooked elbow macaroni, rinsed and drained

In a large skillet sprayed with butter-flavored cooking spray, sauté onion and frankfurters for about 5 minutes. Stir in tomato sauce, bacon bits, Splenda, and mustard. Add pinto beans and macaroni. Mix well to combine. Lower heat and simmer for 5 minutes or until heated through, stirring occasionally.

HINT: Usually ⅔ cup uncooked elbow macaroni cooks to about 1 cup.

Each serving equals:

HE: 2½ Protein • 1¼ Vegetable • ½ Bread •
15 Optional Calories

---

207 Calories • 3 gm Fat • 15 gm Protein •
30 gm Carbohydrate • 996 mg Sodium •
48 mg Calcium • 5 gm Fiber

DIABETIC EXCHANGES: 2 Meat • 1½ Starch • 1 Vegetable

Picnic Casserole

There's nothing more enjoyable than pulling off the road at a pretty picnic area and setting your table with a hot and tasty main dish that everyone will love. Don't forget to let it set before serving—otherwise, it'll likely be too soupy to serve.   ☻   Serves 4

2 full cups (12 ounces) diced cooked potatoes
8 ounces Healthy Choice 97% fat-free frankfurters, diced
1/2 cup frozen peas, thawed
1 (10¾-ounce) can Healthy Request Cream of Mushroom Soup
1/4 cup fat-free milk
1 tablespoon prepared yellow mustard
2 teaspoons dried onion flakes
1/3 cup (1½ ounces) shredded Kraft reduced-fat Cheddar cheese

Preheat oven to 350 degrees. Spray an 8-by-8-inch baking dish with butter-flavored cooking spray. In a large bowl, combine potatoes, frankfurters, and peas. Add mushroom soup, milk, mustard, and onion flakes. Mix gently to combine. Spread mixture into prepared baking dish. Bake for 30 minutes. Evenly sprinkle Cheddar cheese over top. Continue baking for 10 minutes. Place baking dish on a wire rack and let set for 5 minutes. Divide into 4 servings.

HINT: Thaw peas by placing in a colander and rinsing under hot water for 1 minute.

Each serving equals:

HE: 1¾ Protein • 1 Bread • ½ Slider •
5 Optional Calories

233 Calories • 5 gm Fat • 15 gm Protein •
32 gm Carbohydrate • 984 mg Sodium •
163 mg Calcium • 2 gm Fiber

DIABETIC EXCHANGES: 1½ Meat •
1½ Starch/Carbohydrate

Layered Scalloped Potatoes and Ham

My kids always loved scalloped potatoes, so I made them often when they were growing up. Now that they have families of their own, they still love creamy suppers like this ham-and-potatoes version topped with fragrant cheese. ● Serves 4

> 3 cups (15 ounces) peeled and thinly sliced raw potatoes
> ½ cup chopped onion
> 1 (5-ounce) can Hormel lean ham, packed in water, drained and flaked
> ⅓ cup Carnation Nonfat Dry Milk Powder
> ⅓ cup water
> 1 teaspoon dried parsley flakes
> 1 (10¾-ounce) can Healthy Request Cream of Broccoli or Celery Soup
> ¼ cup (¾ ounce) Kraft Reduced Fat Parmesan Style Grated Topping

Preheat oven to 350 degrees. In an 8-by-8-inch baking dish sprayed with butter-flavored cooking spray, layer potatoes, onion, and ham. In a medium bowl, combine dry milk powder, water, parsley flakes, and soup. Evenly spoon mixture over ham. Sprinkle Parmesan cheese evenly over top. Cover and bake for 45 minutes. Uncover and continue baking for 10 to 15 minutes. Place baking dish on a wire rack and let set for 5 minutes. Divide into 4 servings.

Each serving equals:

HE: 1¾ Protein • 1 Bread • ¼ Fat-Free Milk • ¼ Vegetable • ½ Slider • 1 Optional Calorie

192 Calories • 4 gm Fat • 11 gm Protein • 28 gm Carbohydrate • 868 mg Sodium • 134 mg Calcium • 2 gm Fiber

DIABETIC EXCHANGES: 2 Meat • 1½ Starch/Carbohydrate

Skillet Scalloped Cabbage and Ham

This supper-in-a-skillet tastes and looks like you fussed over a hot stove for ages, but its one-pot ease and its cheesy goodness should make it a top-ten-winner on your menu!

○ Serves 4 (1 cup)

> 1 full cup (6 ounces) diced Dubuque 97% fat-free ham or any
>   extra-lean ham
> ½ cup chopped onion
> 3 cups shredded cabbage
> 1 (2.5-ounce) jar sliced mushrooms, drained
> ½ cup water
> 1 (10¾-ounce) can Healthy Request Cream of Mushroom Soup
> ¾ cup (3 ounces) shredded Kraft reduced-fat Cheddar cheese

In a large skillet sprayed with butter-flavored cooking spray, sauté ham and onion for about 5 minutes. Stir in cabbage, mushrooms, and water. Lower heat, cover, and simmer for 15 minutes. Add mushroom soup and Cheddar cheese. Mix well to combine. Continue simmering, uncovered, for 5 to 6 minutes or until cheese is melted, stirring often.

Each serving equals:

HE: 2 Protein • 1¼ Vegetable • ½ Slider •
1 Optional Calorie

---

170 Calories • 6 gm Fat • 15 gm Protein •
14 gm Carbohydrate • 903 mg Sodium •
238 mg Calcium • 2 gm Fiber

DIABETIC EXCHANGES: 2 Meat • 1 Vegetable •
½ Starch/Carbohydrate

Reuben Rice Casserole

I'm not sure who the original "Reuben" was, but my guess is that he was a well-loved man whose wife combined his favorite foods into the nearly perfect sandwich! Well, sometimes you'd rather serve a hot meal instead, so here are all those great flavors in one sizzling dish. ○ Serves 4

> 2 cups cooked rice
> 1 (8-ounce) can sauerkraut, well drained
> 2 (2.5-ounce) packages Carl Buddig 90% lean corned beef, shredded
> ½ cup Kraft Fat Free Thousand Island Dressing
> 2 tablespoons Kraft fat-free mayonnaise
> 1 cup peeled and chopped fresh tomatoes
> 4 (¾-ounce) slices Kraft reduced-fat Swiss cheese

Preheat oven to 350 degrees. Spray an 8-by-8-inch baking dish with butter-flavored cooking spray. In a large bowl, combine rice, sauerkraut, and corned beef. Add Thousand Island dressing and mayonnaise. Mix well to combine. Spread mixture into prepared baking dish. Evenly sprinkle tomatoes over rice mixture. Arrange Swiss cheese slices over top. Bake for 30 to 35 minutes or until hot and bubbly. Place baking dish on a wire rack and let set for 5 minutes. Divide into 4 servings.

HINT: Usually 1⅓ cups uncooked instant rice cooks to about 2 cups.

Each serving equals:

HE: 2¼ Protein • 1 Bread • 1 Vegetable • ½ Slider •
15 Optional Calories

263 Calories • 7 gm Fat • 16 gm Protein •
34 gm Carbohydrate • 929 mg Sodium •
198 mg Calcium • 2 gm Fiber

DIABETIC EXCHANGES: 2 Meat • 1½ Starch • 1 Vegetable

Shortcut Corned Beef Stew

Now that it's possible to buy good-tasting corned beef just about everywhere, a quickie stew that stars this savory meat is not only possible, it's a great standard to have in your repertoire. It's also a good way to use up leftover potatoes if you like.

☉ Serves 4 (1½ cups)

½ cup chopped onion
1 cup chopped celery
1½ cups (8 ounces) diced cooked potatoes
1 (16-ounce) can sliced carrots, rinsed and drained
1 (14½-ounce) can stewed tomatoes, coarsely chopped and
     undrained
1 teaspoon dried parsley flakes
⅛ teaspoon black pepper
2 (2.5-ounce) packages sliced Carl Buddig 90% lean corned beef,
     shredded

In a large skillet sprayed with butter-flavored cooking spray, sauté onion and celery for 10 minutes or until tender. Stir in potatoes, carrots, undrained stewed tomatoes, parsley flakes, and black pepper. Add corned beef. Mix well to combine. Lower heat, cover, and simmer for 10 minutes or until mixture is heated through and vegetables are tender, stirring occasionally.

Each serving equals:

HE: 2½ Vegetable • 1¼ Protein • ½ Bread

142 Calories • 2 gm Fat • 9 gm Protein •
22 gm Carbohydrate • 838 mg Sodium •
92 mg Calcium • 4 gm Fiber

DIABETIC EXCHANGES: 2 Vegetable • 1 Meat • 1 Starch

Kielbasa Supper Skillet

If you've never tasted this popular Polish sausage, be glad that there is a healthy version of it just waiting for you to try! Heartier than hot dogs, kielbasa packs so much flavor into every bite, you'll be ready to rise from the table and polka! ☺ Serves 4 (1 full cup)

16 ounces Healthy Choice 97% lean kielbasa sausage,
  cut into ½-inch pieces
2 cups shredded cabbage
2 cups (10 ounces) unpeeled and sliced raw potatoes
1 cup chopped onion
¾ cup water
2 teaspoons dried parsley flakes
⅛ teaspoon black pepper

In a large skillet sprayed with butter-flavored cooking spray, sauté sausage for 5 minutes. Stir in cabbage, potatoes, onion, and water. Add parsley flakes and black pepper. Mix well to combine. Lower heat, cover, and simmer for 30 minutes or until vegetables are tender, stirring occasionally.

Each serving equals:

HE: 3 Protein • 1 Vegetable • ½ Bread

253 Calories • 9 gm Fat • 21 gm Protein •
22 gm Carbohydrate • 815 mg Sodium •
36 mg Calcium • 3 gm Fiber

DIABETIC EXCHANGES: 3 Meat • 1 Vegetable • 1 Starch

Speedy Desserts

Now that I've seen nearly all of the fifty states from the kitchen window of our motor home or the passenger seat of our car, I can say without reservation that the best part of living "on the go" is meeting wonderful people from just about everywhere. Whether you're visiting with new friends or sharing memories with old ones, you're likely to sit down over coffee and a delectable dessert. I've even been able to fix the perfect pie in just minutes when someone stops by. And I'm rarely without pudding in the fridge and freshly made cookies cooling on the counter!

What a comfort to know that you can whip up something scrumptious to serve your guests in just minutes—especially treats like **Razzle Dazzle Banana Cream Pie** or **Chocolate Velvet Ribbon Dessert**! Even when you're only feeding the family, you can quickly raise road-weary spirits with **Triple Treat Chocolate Cake Brownies** (maybe drizzled with a little **Hot Peanut Butter Fudge Sauce!**) or make Anytown, USA, feel like home with an old-fashioned delight like **Cinnamon Cherry Cobbler**. And if you've got a special occasion—a birthday or anniversary—that rings in while you're far away, celebrate being together with **Fantastic Fruit Cocktail Cake** or (my family's favorite) some **Chocolate Peppermint Cheesecake**!

Speedy Desserts

Hot Peanut Butter Fudge Sauce

Forget those high-fat and expensive gourmet ice creams that cost your pocketbook as much as they do your health. Instead, choose a healthy low-fat or fat-free ice cream or yogurt, and drizzle this out-of-this-world sauce over the top. Paradise for peanut butter lovers!

◐ Serves 6 (¼ cup)

> 1 (4-serving) package JELL-O sugar-free chocolate cook-and-serve
>   pudding mix
> ⅔ cup Carnation Nonfat Dry Milk Powder
> 1½ cups water
> 6 tablespoons Peter Pan reduced-fat creamy peanut butter
> 1 teaspoon vanilla extract

In a medium saucepan, combine dry pudding mix, dry milk powder, and water. Cook over medium heat until mixture thickens and starts to boil, stirring constantly using a wire whisk. Remove from heat. Add peanut butter and vanilla extract. Mix well to combine. Spoon hot sauce over ice cream or cake.

HINT: Leftovers reheat beautifully in the microwave.

Each serving equals:

HE: 1 Protein • 1 Fat • ⅓ Fat-Free Milk •
13 Optional Calories

---

129 Calories • 5 gm Fat • 8 gm Protein •
13 gm Carbohydrate • 204 mg Sodium •
106 mg Calcium • 1 gm Fiber

DIABETIC EXCHANGES: 1 Starch/Carbohydrate •
½ Meat • ½ Fat

Magic Micro Walnut Fudge

I'm convinced that one of the best uses for your microwave is to make the most fantastic fudge. Here's a version that is so spectacularly good, it'll disappear before you can say, "Abracadabra!"

● Serves 16 (2 each)

> 1⅓ cups Carnation Nonfat Dry Milk Powder
> ½ cup water
> 2¼ cups Splenda Granular ☆
> 1½ cups mini chocolate chips
> 6 squares unsweetened baking chocolate
> 1 tablespoon + 1 teaspoon vanilla extract
> ½ cup (2 ounces) chopped walnuts

In a microwave-safe 8-cup measuring cup, combine dry milk powder and water. Microwave on HIGH (100% power) for 45 to 60 seconds or until mixture is almost boiling. Stir in ½ cup Splenda. Cover and refrigerate for at least 2 hours. Stir chocolate chips, baking chocolate, and remaining 1¾ cups Splenda into milk mixture. Microwave on HIGH for 2 minutes, stirring after 1 minute. Add vanilla extract and walnuts. Mix well to combine. Spray a 9-by-9-inch cake pan with butter-flavored cooking spray. Evenly spread fudge mixture into prepared cake pan. Refrigerate for at least 2 hours. Cut into 32 pieces.

Each serving equals:

> HE: 1 Fat • ¼ Fat-Free Milk • 1 Slider •
> 18 Optional Calories
> ───────────────────────────────
> 169 Calories • 9 gm Fat • 5 gm Protein •
> 17 gm Carbohydrate • 34 mg Sodium •
> 86 mg Calcium • 2 gm Fiber
> ───────────────────────────────
> DIABETIC EXCHANGES: 1½ Fat • 1 Starch/Carbohydrate

Apple Spice Hermits

I don't know for sure where these spicy-fruity cookies got their name, but I have an idea. As soon as you nibble on one, you're ready to grab the rest and head for a cave to enjoy them in private! (Now, don't be that way—it's always best to share.)

❂ Serves 12 (3 each)

> 1 cup Bisquick Reduced Fat Baking Mix
> 2/3 cup quick oats
> 1/2 cup Splenda Granular
> 1/2 teaspoon baking powder
> 1 teaspoon apple pie spice
> 1/2 cup Musselman's "No Sugar Added" Applesauce
> 1 tablespoon + 1 teaspoon I Can't Believe It's Not Butter! Light
>   Margarine
> 1/4 cup Land O Lakes no-fat sour cream
> 1 egg or equivalent in egg substitute
> 1 1/2 cups (3 small) cored, peeled, and chopped apples
> 1/2 cup raisins
> 1/4 cup chopped walnuts

Preheat oven to 375 degrees. Spray 3 baking sheets with butter-flavored cooking spray. In a large bowl, combine baking mix, oats, Splenda, baking powder, and apple pie spice. In a small bowl, combine applesauce, margarine, sour cream, and egg. Add liquid mixture to dry mixture. Mix gently to combine. Fold in apples, raisins, and walnuts. Drop by spoonful onto prepared baking sheets to form 36 cookies. Spray bottom of a glass with butter-flavored cooking spray and lightly flatten cookies. Bake for 8 to 10 minutes or until golden brown. Place cookies on wire racks and allow to cool.

Each serving equals:

HE: 3/4 Fat • 2/3 Bread • 2/3 Fruit • 1/3 Protein •
9 Optional Calories

119 Calories • 3 gm Fat • 3 gm Protein •
20 gm Carbohydrate • 164 mg Sodium •
41 mg Calcium • 1 gm Fiber

DIABETIC EXCHANGES: 1 Starch • 1/2 Fruit • 1/2 Fat

Peanut Butter Candy Cookies

Mmm-mm good—that's what everyone said when we tested these cookies that are so yummy even candy lovers will choose them instead! ☻ Serves 8 (4 each)

½ cup Peter Pan reduced-fat peanut butter
½ cup Splenda Granular
⅔ cup Carnation Nonfat Dry Milk Powder
¼ cup water
2½ cups cornflakes

Preheat oven to 375 degrees. In a large bowl, combine peanut butter, Splenda, dry milk powder, and water until smooth. Add cornflakes. Mix well until thoroughly blended. Using clean hands, form into 32 balls. Place balls on ungreased baking sheet and flatten each with the bottom of a glass sprayed with butter-flavored cooking spray. Bake for 5 to 6 minutes or until browned. Place cookies on a wire rack and allow to cool.

Each serving equals:

HE: 1 Protein • 1 Fat • ½ Bread • ¼ Fat-Free Milk •
6 Optional Calories

203 Calories • 7 gm Fat • 10 gm Protein •
25 gm Carbohydrate • 336 mg Sodium •
109 mg Calcium • 2 gm Fiber

DIABETIC EXCHANGES: 1½ Starch/Carbohydrate •
½ Meat • ½ Fat

Triple Treat Chocolate
Cake Brownies

Every healthy cook needs at least one brilliant brownie recipe, and this might be the one that wins your heart forever. Featuring three bursts of chocolate flavor, plus sour cream and nuts, these brownies will produce happy cries of "Yes, yes, yes!"   ☻   Serves 12 (2 each)

¼ cup + 1 tablespoon I Can't
   Believe It's Not Butter!
   Light Margarine ☆
¼ cup + 2 tablespoons Land O
   Lakes no-fat sour cream ☆
1 egg or equivalent in egg
   substitute
½ cup water

2½ teaspoons vanilla extract ☆
1¾ cups Splenda Granular ☆
1 cup + 2 tablespoons Bisquick
   Reduced Fat Baking Mix
¼ cup unsweetened cocoa
¼ cup chopped walnuts ☆
¼ cup mini chocolate chips
1 square unsweetened chocolate

Preheat oven to 350 degrees. Spray an 11-by-7-inch biscuit pan with butter-flavored cooking spray. In a large bowl, combine ¼ cup margarine, ¼ cup sour cream, and egg. Stir in water, 1½ teaspoons vanilla extract, and ¾ cup Splenda. Add baking mix and cocoa. Mix well to combine. Fold in 3 tablespoons walnuts and chocolate chips. Evenly spread batter in prepared biscuit pan. Sprinkle with remaining walnuts. Bake for 15 to 18 minutes. Place biscuit pan on a wire rack. Meanwhile, in a small saucepan sprayed with butter-flavored cooking spray, melt remaining 1 tablespoon margarine, remaining 2 tablespoons sour cream, and chocolate square over low heat. Stir in remaining 1 teaspoon vanilla extract and remaining 1 cup Splenda. Remove from heat. Drizzle warm mixture evenly over warm brownies. Continue cooling for at least 15 minutes. Cut into 24 pieces.

Each serving equals:

HE: ⅔ Fat • ½ Bread • ¾ Slider

161 Calories • 9 gm Fat • 3 gm Protein •
17 gm Carbohydrate • 254 mg Sodium •
38 mg Calcium • 1 gm Fiber

DIABETIC EXCHANGES: 1½ Fat • 1 Starch/Carbohydrate

Vanilla Fruit Pudding

Some people call vanilla the plainest flavor there is, but those folks never tasted this version of vanilla! With a bit of extract, all that sweet fruit, and the extra *ooomph* added by the dry milk powder, this recipe is a winner!   ☻   Serves 4

> 1 (4-serving) package JELL-O sugar-free vanilla cook-and-serve
>   pudding mix
> ⅔ cup Carnation Nonfat Dry Milk Powder
> 1 (16-ounce) can fruit cocktail, packed in fruit juice, drained and
>   ½ cup liquid reserved
> 1 cup water
> 1 teaspoon vanilla extract

In a medium saucepan, combine dry pudding mix, dry milk powder, reserved fruit cocktail liquid, and water. Cook over medium heat until mixture thickens and starts to boil, stirring constantly. Remove from heat. Stir in vanilla extract and fruit cocktail. Spoon mixture into 4 dessert dishes. Refrigerate for at least 30 minutes.

Each serving equals:

HE: 1 Fruit • ½ Fat-Free Milk • ¼ Slider

116 Calories • 0 gm Fat • 4 gm Protein •
25 gm Carbohydrate • 182 mg Sodium •
159 mg Calcium • 1 gm Fiber

DIABETIC EXCHANGES: 1 Fruit • ½ Fat-Free Milk

Heavenly Lemon Cream

After you've spent a little while admiring those puffy clouds from your lawn chair, it's time for a dessert as luscious as a sunny summer sky. Hear those angels singing? They've just dined on this glorious dish. ☻ Serves 4

> 1 (4-serving) package JELL-O sugar-free instant vanilla pudding mix
> 1 (4-serving) package JELL-O sugar-free lemon gelatin
> ⅔ cup Carnation Nonfat Dry Milk Powder
> 1 cup Diet Mountain Dew
> ½ cup Land O Lakes no-fat sour cream
> ½ cup Cool Whip Free

In a large bowl, combine dry pudding mix, dry gelatin, dry milk powder, and Diet Mountain Dew. Mix well using a wire whisk. Blend in sour cream and Cool Whip Free. Evenly spoon mixture into 4 dessert dishes. Refrigerate for at least 15 minutes.

Each serving equals:

HE: ½ Fat-Free Milk • 1 Slider • 5 Optional Calories

---

104 Calories • 0 gm Fat • 6 gm Protein •
20 gm Carbohydrate • 282 mg Sodium •
170 mg Calcium • 0 gm Fiber

DIABETIC EXCHANGES: 1 Starch/Carbohydrate •
½ Fat-Free Milk

Citrus Pudding

It's light, it's refreshing, and it even delivers a terrific wallop of vitamin C. This lemon-orange delight is creamy and oh-so-sweet.

● Serves 4

> 1 (4-serving) package JELL-O sugar-free instant vanilla pudding
> mix
> 1 (4-serving) package JELL-O sugar-free lemon gelatin
> ⅔ cup Carnation Nonfat Dry Milk Powder
> 1¼ cups water
> ½ cup Cool Whip Free
> 1 (11-ounce) can mandarin oranges, rinsed and drained

In a large bowl, combine dry pudding mix, dry gelatin, and dry milk powder. Add water. Mix well using a wire whisk. Blend in Cool Whip Free. Gently stir in mandarin oranges. Evenly spoon mixture into 4 dessert dishes. Refrigerate for at least 15 minutes.

Each serving equals:

HE: ½ Fat-Free Milk • ½ Fruit • ½ Slider •
10 Optional Calories

---

108 Calories • 0 gm Fat • 4 gm Protein •
23 gm Carbohydrate • 192 mg Sodium •
150 mg Calcium • 0 gm Fiber

DIABETIC EXCHANGES: ½ Fat-Free Milk • ½ Fruit •
½ Starch/Carbohydrate

Tutti-Frutti Pudding Treats

If you're one of those dessert lovers who want it all, then tutti-frutti might be the perfect flavor for you! There's just something so much fun about finding goodies in your pudding.   ☻   Serves 4

> 1 (4-serving) package JELL-O sugar-free instant vanilla pudding mix
> ⅔ cup Carnation Nonfat Dry Milk Powder
> 1 cup water
> 1 (8-ounce) can crushed pineapple, packed in fruit juice, undrained
> ¼ cup Cool Whip Free
> 2 tablespoons (½ ounce) chopped pecans
> ¼ cup miniature marshmallows
> 4 maraschino cherries, quartered

In a large bowl, combine dry pudding mix, dry milk powder, water, and undrained pineapple. Mix well using a wire whisk. Blend in Cool Whip Free. Add pecans, marshmallows, and cherries. Mix gently to combine. Evenly spoon mixture into 4 dessert dishes. Refrigerate for at least 30 minutes.

Each serving equals:

HE: ½ Fat-Free Milk • ½ Fruit • ½ Fat • ½ Slider • 9 Optional Calories

---

150 Calories • 2 gm Fat • 4 gm Protein • 29 gm Carbohydrate • 396 mg Sodium • 148 mg Calcium • 1 gm Fiber

---

DIABETIC EXCHANGES: 1 Starch/Carbohydrate • ½ Fat-Free Milk • ½ Fruit • ½ Fat

Coconut Pecan Pudding Treats

Some people prefer their puddings creamy and free of added textures, but I know many who prefer to discover little treasures in each bite! Here, the surprises include delicious flaked coconut and bits of my favorite nut, the pecan.   ❂   Serves 4

> 1 (4-serving) package JELL-O sugar-free instant vanilla pudding
>   mix
> ⅔ cup Carnation Nonfat Dry Milk Powder
> 1⅓ cups water
> ½ cup Cool Whip Free
> 1 teaspoon coconut extract
> 2 tablespoons chopped pecans
> 2 tablespoons flaked coconut

In a medium bowl, combine dry pudding mix, dry milk powder, and water. Mix well using a wire whisk. Blend in Cool Whip Free and coconut extract. Evenly spoon mixture into 4 dessert dishes. Sprinkle 1½ teaspoons pecans and coconut over top of each. Refrigerate for at least 15 minutes.

Each serving equals:

HE: ½ Fat-Free Milk • ½ Fat • ½ Slider •
8 Optional Calories

---

107 Calories • 3 gm Fat • 4 gm Protein •
16 gm Carbohydrate • 403 mg Sodium •
153 mg Calcium • 0 gm Fiber

DIABETIC EXCHANGES: ½ Fat-Free Milk • ½ Fat •
½ Starch/Carbohydrate

Creamy Peach Pudding

My daughter, Becky, is the family peach enthusiast, and I know this delectable dessert would please her in every way. Even if peaches are in season, follow the recipe's instructions to use canned peaches— they just work better in this dish.   ☻   Serves 4

> 1 (4-serving) package JELL-O sugar-free instant vanilla pudding mix
> ⅔ cup Carnation Nonfat Dry Milk Powder
> 1 (16-ounce) can sliced peaches, packed in fruit juice, drained and ⅓ cup liquid reserved
> 1 cup water
> ⅓ cup Land O Lakes no-fat sour cream
> ¼ teaspoon ground nutmeg

In a large bowl, combine dry pudding mix and dry milk powder. Add reserved peach liquid and water. Mix well using a wire whisk. Blend in sour cream and nutmeg. Spoon about ¼ cup pudding mixture into 4 tall dessert dishes. Evenly divide peaches between 4 dishes. Evenly spoon about ¼ cup remaining pudding mixture over each. Refrigerate for at least 30 minutes.

Each serving equals:

HE: 1 Fruit • ½ Fat-Free Milk • ½ Slider • 5 Optional Calories

---

148 Calories • 0 gm Fat • 6 gm Protein •
31 gm Carbohydrate • 423 mg Sodium •
184 mg Calcium • 2 gm Fiber

DIABETIC EXCHANGES: 1 Fruit • ½ Fat-Free Milk • ½ Starch/Carbohydrate

Applesauce Raisin Cream Pudding

When my friend Barbara was growing up, her mom stirred applesauce and raisins into her oatmeal, so when she saw this recipe, she knew right away she had to try it. Her reaction: "Ooooohhhhhhh, that's good!" ❂ Serves 4

1 (4-serving) package JELL-O sugar-free instant vanilla pudding mix
⅔ cup Carnation Nonfat Dry Milk Powder
1 teaspoon apple pie spice
1 cup Musselman's "No Sugar Added" Applesauce
½ cup water
¼ cup raisins
¼ cup Cool Whip Lite

In a medium bowl, combine dry pudding mix, dry milk powder, and apple pie spice. Add applesauce and water. Mix well using a wire whisk. Blend in raisins and Cool Whip Lite. Evenly spoon mixture into 4 dessert dishes. Refrigerate for at least 30 minutes.

Each serving equals:

HE: 1 Fruit • ½ Fat-Free Milk • ¼ Slider •
15 Optional Calories

124 Calories • 0 gm Fat • 4 gm Protein •
27 gm Carbohydrate • 394 mg Sodium •
156 mg Calcium • 1 gm Fiber

DIABETIC EXCHANGES: 1 Fruit • ½ Fat-Free Milk

Special Banana Pudding

It's cool and creamy, soft and sweet—and brimming with bits of banana! The cinnamon graham crackers deliver a spicy wallop of flavor that is hard to resist. ☻   Serves 6

> 1 (4-serving) package JELL-O sugar-free instant vanilla pudding
>   mix
> ⅔ cup Carnation Nonfat Dry Milk Powder
> 1½ cups water
> ¾ cup plain fat-free yogurt
> ¾ cup Cool Whip Free
> 1 teaspoon vanilla extract
> 2 cups (2 medium) diced bananas
> 12 (2½-inch) cinnamon graham crackers, coarsely broken

In a large bowl, combine dry pudding mix, dry milk powder, and water. Mix well using a wire whisk. Blend in yogurt, Cool Whip Free, and vanilla extract. Add bananas. Mix gently to combine. Gently fold in graham cracker pieces. Evenly spoon mixture into 6 dessert dishes. Refrigerate for at least 15 minutes.

Each serving equals:

HE: ⅔ Bread • ⅔ Fruit • ½ Fat-Free Milk • ¼ Slider •
12 Optional Calories

---

178 Calories • 2 gm Fat • 6 gm Protein •
34 gm Carbohydrate • 375 mg Sodium •
167 mg Calcium • 2 gm Fiber

DIABETIC EXCHANGES: 1 Starch • ½ Fruit •
½ Fat-Free Milk

Graham Cracker Banana Pudding

After a long, long, long day on the road, you'll win the hearts of your little ones when you serve this child-pleasing dish. I'm not sure why graham crackers and bananas remind us all of childhood, but they do! ☻ Serves 4

> 1 (4-serving) package JELL-O sugar-free vanilla cook-and-serve pudding mix
> 2 tablespoons Splenda Granular
> 2 cups fat-free milk
> 1 teaspoon vanilla extract
> 1/2 cup purchased graham cracker crumbs or 9 (2 1/2-inch) graham cracker squares, made into crumbs
> 2 cups (2 medium) diced bananas
> 1/4 cup Cool Whip Lite
> 1 tablespoon chopped pecans

In a medium saucepan, combine dry pudding mix, Splenda, and milk. Cook over medium heat until mixture thickens and starts to boil, stirring constantly. Remove from heat. Add vanilla extract and graham cracker crumbs. Mix gently to combine. Fold in bananas. Evenly spoon mixture into 4 dessert dishes. Refrigerate for at least 30 minutes. Just before serving, top each with 1 tablespoon Cool Whip Lite and 3/4 teaspoon pecans.

HINT: To prevent bananas from turning brown, mix with 1 teaspoon lemon juice or sprinkle with Fruit Fresh.

Each serving equals:

HE: 1 Fruit • 3/4 Bread • 1/2 Fat-Free Milk • 1/4 Fat • 1/4 Slider • 13 Optional Calories

212 Calories • 4 gm Fat • 6 gm Protein • 38 gm Carbohydrate • 269 mg Sodium • 160 mg Calcium • 2 gm Fiber

DIABETIC EXCHANGES: 1 Fruit • 1 Starch • 1/2 Fat-Free Milk

Chocolate Orange Mousse

What a winning combination this is—dark fudge and sunny citrus! This is oh-so-good—and good for you, too!   ☻   Serves 4

> 1 (4-serving) package JELL-O sugar-free instant chocolate fudge pudding mix
> ⅔ cup Carnation Nonfat Dry Milk Powder
> 1 cup unsweetened orange juice
> ½ cup Cool Whip Free

In a large bowl, combine dry pudding mix, dry milk powder, and orange juice. Mix well using a wire whisk. Blend in Cool Whip Free. Evenly spoon mixture into 4 dessert dishes. Refrigerate for at least 15 minutes.

Each serving equals:

HE: ½ Fat-Free Milk • ½ Fruit • ½ Slider • 10 Optional Calories

112 Calories • 0 gm Fat • 5 gm Protein • 23 gm Carbohydrate • 398 mg Sodium • 143 mg Calcium • 0 gm Fiber

DIABETIC EXCHANGES: ½ Fat-Free Milk • ½ Fruit • ½ Starch/Carbohydrate

Lemon-Pineapple Rice Pudding

Why settle for plain rice pudding when you can celebrate with so much tangy citrus taste? The Diet Mountain Dew adds yet one more luscious layer of lemon.   ● Serves 6

1 (4-serving) package JELL-O sugar-free instant vanilla pudding
    mix
1 (4-serving) package JELL-O sugar-free lemon gelatin
⅔ cup Carnation Nonfat Dry Milk Powder
1 (8-ounce) can crushed pineapple, packed in fruit juice, undrained
1 cup Diet Mountain Dew
½ cup Cool Whip Lite
1½ cups cold cooked rice

In a large bowl, combine dry pudding mix, dry gelatin, dry milk powder, undrained pineapple, and Diet Mountain Dew. Mix well using a wire whisk. Blend in Cool Whip Lite. Add rice. Mix gently to combine. Evenly spoon mixture into 6 dessert dishes. Refrigerate for at least 15 minutes.

HINT: Usually 1 cup uncooked instant rice cooks to about 1½ cups.

Each serving equals:

HE: ½ Bread • ⅓ Fat-Free Milk • ⅓ Fruit •
¼ Slider • 17 Optional Calories

109 Calories • 1 gm Fat • 4 gm Protein •
21 gm Carbohydrate • 270 mg Sodium •
108 mg Calcium • 1 gm Fiber

DIABETIC EXCHANGES: 1½ Starch/Carbohydrate

Chocolate–Peanut Butter Dessert

Peanuts *and* peanut butter—isn't that just a little too decadent? Oh, yes, indeed! It only takes a little of each to make this treat irresistible.

● Serves 6

> 1 (4-serving) package JELL-O sugar-free chocolate cook-and-serve pudding mix
> ⅔ cup Carnation Nonfat Dry Milk Powder
> 1¾ cups water
> 2 tablespoons Peter Pan reduced-fat peanut butter
> 1 teaspoon vanilla extract
> ¼ cup (1 ounce) chopped dry-roasted peanuts
> ¾ cup Cool Whip Free
> 9 (2½-inch) peanut butter or regular graham crackers, broken into large pieces

In a large saucepan, combine dry pudding mix, dry milk powder, and water. Cook over medium heat until mixture thickens and starts to boil, stirring often. Add peanut butter and vanilla extract. Mix well using a wire whisk. Spoon mixture into a large bowl. Stir in peanuts. Place bowl on a wire rack and allow to cool for 30 minutes, stirring occasionally. Fold in Cool Whip Free and graham cracker pieces. Evenly spoon mixture into 6 dessert dishes. Refrigerate for at least 15 minutes.

Each serving equals:

HE: ⅔ Fat • ½ Bread • ½ Protein • ⅓ Fat-Free Milk • ½ Slider

145 Calories • 5 gm Fat • 6 gm Protein • 19 gm Carbohydrate • 182 mg Sodium • 98 mg Calcium • 1 gm Fiber

DIABETIC EXCHANGES: 1 Starch/Carbohydrate • 1 Fat • ½ Meat

Chocolate Velvet Ribbon Dessert

You've got to love these layers of rich and creamy chocolate, or you can't call yourself a true chocoholic! As long as you've got pudding and Cool Whip on hand, you're always good to go.   ❤   Serves 8

12 (2½-inch) chocolate graham
    cracker squares ☆
1 (4-serving) package JELL-O
    sugar-free instant
    chocolate fudge pudding
    mix
2 cups Carnation Nonfat Dry
    Milk Powder ☆

3¼ cups water ☆
1 (4-serving) package JELL-O
    sugar-free instant
    chocolate pudding mix
1 cup Cool Whip Free ☆
1 (4-serving) package JELL-O
    sugar-free instant white
    chocolate pudding mix

Arrange 9 graham crackers in a 9-by-9-inch cake pan, breaking as necessary to fit. In a large bowl, combine dry chocolate fudge pudding mix, ⅔ cup dry milk powder, and 1¼ cups water. Mix well using a wire whisk. Carefully spoon mixture evenly over crackers. Refrigerate while preparing next layer. In same bowl, combine dry chocolate pudding mix, another ⅔ cup dry milk powder, and 1 cup water. Mix well, using a wire whisk. Blend in ½ cup Cool Whip Free. Spread mixture evenly over set chocolate fudge layer. Refrigerate while preparing next layer. In a clean large bowl, combine dry white chocolate pudding mix, remaining ⅔ cup dry milk powder, and remaining 1 cup water. Mix well using a clean wire whisk. Blend in remaining ½ cup Cool Whip Free. Spread mixture evenly over chocolate layer. Crush remaining 3 graham crackers and evenly sprinkle crumbs over top. Cover and refrigerate for at least 2 hours. Cut into 8 servings.

HINT: A self-seal sandwich bag works great for crushing graham
    crackers.

Each serving equals:

HE: ¾ Fat-Free Milk • ½ Bread • ¾ Slider •
5 Optional Calories

145 Calories • 1 gm Fat • 7 gm Protein •
27 gm Carbohydrate • 627 mg Sodium •
209 mg Calcium • 0 gm Fiber

DIABETIC EXCHANGES: 1½ Starch/Carbohydrate •
½ Fat-Free Milk

Chocolate–Peanut Butter Bread Pudding

Instead of succumbing to high-calorie peanut butter cups, try this scrumptious way of getting your chocolate–peanut butter fix! I bet you'll be surprised and delighted by how rich this recipe tastes.

☺ Serves 6

1 (4-serving) package JELL-O sugar-free chocolate cook-and-serve pudding mix
3 cups fat-free milk
¼ cup Peter Pan reduced-fat peanut butter
¼ cup Splenda Granular
1 teaspoon vanilla extract
12 slices reduced-calorie white bread, torn into pieces
3 tablespoons mini chocolate chips

Preheat oven to 350 degrees. Spray an 8-by-8-inch baking dish with butter-flavored cooking spray. In a large saucepan, combine dry pudding mix and milk. Cook over medium heat until mixture starts to thicken and begins to boil, stirring often. Remove from heat. Stir in peanut butter, Splenda, and vanilla extract. Add bread pieces. Mix gently to combine. Spread mixture evenly into prepared baking dish. Evenly sprinkle chocolate chips over top. Bake for 30 minutes. Place baking dish on a wire rack and let set for 5 minutes. Divide into 6 servings.

Each serving equals:

HE: 1 Bread • ⅔ Protein • ⅔ Fat • ½ Fat-Free Milk • ¼ Slider • 16 Optional Calories

---

246 Calories • 6 gm Fat • 12 gm Protein •
36 mg Carbohydrate • 452 mg Sodium •
183 mg Calcium • 1 gm Fiber

DIABETIC EXCHANGES: 1 Starch/Carbohydrate • 1 Fat •
½ Meat • ½ Fat-Free Milk

Caribbean Bread Pudding

Maybe this taste treat will be as close as you get to the islands this year, but that's no reason not to put a little Gloria Estefan on the CD player and pretend you're sunning on a white sandy beach. Mm-mm!

♥ Serves 6

4 individual sponge cake dessert cups, broken into large pieces
1 (4-serving) package JELL-O sugar-free vanilla cook-and-serve
  pudding mix
⅔ cup Carnation Nonfat Dry Milk Powder
2 (8-ounce) cans crushed pineapple, packed in fruit juice,
  undrained
1 cup water
1 teaspoon coconut extract
1 teaspoon rum extract
2 tablespoons flaked coconut

Preheat oven to 350 degrees. Spray an 8-by-8-inch baking dish with butter-flavored cooking spray. Evenly arrange sponge cake pieces in prepared baking dish. In a large saucepan, combine dry pudding mix, dry milk powder, undrained pineapple, and water. Cook over medium heat until mixture thickens and starts to boil, stirring often. Remove from heat. Stir in coconut and rum extracts. Pour hot mixture evenly over sponge cake pieces. Evenly sprinkle coconut over top. Bake for 25 to 30 minutes. Place baking dish on a wire rack and let set for 5 minutes. Divide into 6 servings.

Each serving equals:

HE: ¾ Bread • ⅔ Fruit • ⅓ Fat-Free Milk •
18 Optional Calories

138 Calories • 2 gm Fat • 4 gm Protein •
26 gm Carbohydrate • 209 mg Sodium •
119 mg Calcium • 2 gm Fiber

DIABETIC EXCHANGES: 1 Starch/Carbohydrate • ½ Fruit

Pumpkin Pie Pudding Squares

If you've never baked with pumpkin, I'm here to tell you that it makes for super-moist results! Serve these during harvest season for a perfect fit, but they're good all year long. ☺ Serves 8

⅔ cup Carnation Nonfat Dry Milk Powder
1¼ cups water
1 egg, slightly beaten, or equivalent in egg substitute
¾ cup Splenda Granular
1½ teaspoons pumpkin pie spice
½ teaspoon vanilla extract
1 (15-ounce) can Libby's Solid Pack Pumpkin
1 cup Bisquick Reduced Fat Baking Mix

Preheat oven to 350 degrees. Spray an 8-by-12-inch baking dish with butter-flavored cooking spray. In a large bowl, combine dry milk powder and water. Stir in egg, Splenda, pumpkin pie spice, and vanilla extract. Add pumpkin and baking mix. Mix well using a wire whisk. Spread mixture into prepared baking dish. Bake for 45 to 50 minutes or until a toothpick inserted near center comes out clean. Place baking dish on a wire rack and let set for at least 10 minutes. Divide into 8 servings. Serve warm or cold.

Each serving equals:

HE: ⅔ Bread • ½ Vegetable • ¼ Fat-Free Milk • 17 Optional Calories

---

105 Calories • 1 gm Fat • 5 gm Protein •
19 gm Carbohydrate • 215 mg Sodium •
113 mg Calcium • 2 gm Fiber

DIABETIC EXCHANGES: 1½ Starch/Carbohydrate

Fantastic Fruit Cocktail Cake

Here's a clever cook's best friend—a delectable dessert ready in just minutes and prepared from handy ingredients we all keep on our pantry shelves.   ☺   Serves 2

6 tablespoons Bisquick Reduced Fat Baking Mix
⅓ cup Splenda Granular
¼ teaspoon ground cinnamon
2 tablespoons chopped walnuts
1 (8-ounce) can fruit cocktail, packed in fruit juice, undrained
1 egg or equivalent in egg substitute

Preheat oven to 350 degrees. Spray two (12-ounce) custard cups with butter-flavored cooking spray. In a medium bowl, combine baking mix, Splenda, cinnamon, and walnuts. Add undrained fruit cocktail and egg. Mix well to combine. Evenly spoon batter into prepared custard cups. Place filled cups on a baking sheet and bake for 20 to 25 minutes or until a toothpick inserted near center comes out clean. Place custard cups on a wire rack and allow to cool completely.

HINT: Good served with 1 tablespoon Cool Whip Lite but don't forget to count the additional calories.

Each serving equals:

HE: 1 Bread • 1 Fruit • ¾ Protein • ½ Fat •
16 Optional Calories

---

237 Calories • 9 gm Fat • 7 gm Protein •
32 gm Carbohydrate • 298 mg Sodium •
55 mg Calcium • 2 gm Fiber

DIABETIC EXCHANGES: 1 Starch • 1 Fruit • 1 Fat •
½ Meat

Sour Cream Shortcakes

These are wonderfully light and fluffy, perfect for serving with some ruby gems from your garden. When your strawberries are ready to be harvested, treat them (and yourself!) to a perfectly tasty "frame."

● Serves 4

> 3/4 cup Bisquick Reduced Fat Baking Mix
> 2 tablespoons Splenda Granular
> 6 tablespoons Land O Lakes no-fat sour cream
> 1 tablespoon fat-free milk

Preheat oven to 425 degrees. Spray a baking sheet with butter-flavored cooking spray. In a medium bowl, combine baking mix and Splenda. Add sour cream and milk. Mix just until moistened. Using a scant 1/4 cup, pour batter onto prepared baking sheet to form 4 shortcakes. Bake for 10 to 12 minutes or until golden brown.

Each serving equals:

HE: 1 Bread • 1/4 Slider • 3 Optional Calories

101 Calories • 1 gm Fat • 3 gm Protein •
20 gm Carbohydrate • 293 mg Sodium •
47 mg Calcium • 0 gm Fiber

DIABETIC EXCHANGES: 1 Starch

Pecan Delight Dessert Pizza

Never heard of dessert pizza before? I've created quite a few of these, but perhaps never one as tasty as this one! How can you go wrong with pecans and chocolate?　　◐　　Serves 12

1 (11-ounce) can Pillsbury refrigerated French loaf
1 (4-serving) package JELL-O sugar-free vanilla cook-and-serve
    pudding mix
¼ cup Splenda Granular
1½ cups water
2 teaspoons vanilla extract
½ cup (2 ounces) chopped pecans
½ cup mini chocolate chips

Preheat oven to 350 degrees. Spray a rimmed 10-by-15-inch baking sheet with butter-flavored cooking spray. Unroll French loaf and pat evenly into prepared baking sheet. Bake for 8 minutes. Meanwhile, in a medium saucepan, combine dry pudding mix, Splenda, and water. Cook over medium heat until mixture thickens and starts to boil, stirring constantly. Remove from heat. Stir in vanilla extract. Spoon hot mixture evenly over partially baked crust. Evenly sprinkle pecans and chocolate chips over top. Continue baking for 7 to 8 minutes or until crust is golden brown. Place baking sheet on a wire rack and allow to cool completely. Cut into 12 servings.

Each serving equals:

HE: ⅔ Bread • ⅔ Fat • ¼ Slider •
14 Optional Calories

138 Calories • 6 gm Fat • 3 gm Protein •
18 gm Carbohydrate • 202 mg Sodium •
5 mg Calcium • 1 gm Fiber

DIABETIC EXCHANGES: 1 Starch • 1 Fat

Cinnamon Cherry Cobbler

Ever since the father of our country nearly sacrificed his good name for love of cherries (isn't that why he cut down the cherry tree? I wonder!), many others have lost their hearts to this ruby-colored fruit. . . . ☻ Serves 8

> 1 (4-serving) package JELL-O sugar-free vanilla cook-and-serve pudding mix
> 1 (4-serving) package JELL-O sugar-free cherry gelatin
> 1 (16-ounce) can tart red cherries, packed in water, drained, and ½ cup liquid reserved
> ½ cup water
> 1 (8-ounce) can Pillsbury Reduced Fat Crescent Rolls
> 2 tablespoons Splenda Granular
> 1 teaspoon ground cinnamon

In a medium saucepan, combine dry pudding mix, dry gelatin, reserved cherry liquid, water, and cherries. Cook over medium heat until mixture thickens and starts to boil, stirring constantly, being careful not to crush cherries. Remove from heat. Pour mixture into an 8-by-8-inch baking dish. Pat crescent rolls into a rectangle, being sure to seal perforations. In a small bowl, combine Splenda and cinnamon. Evenly sprinkle mixture over rolls. Roll up jelly-roll style. Cut into 16 even slices. Place slices evenly over cherry mixture. Lightly spray tops with butter-flavored cooking spray. Bake in a 375-degree oven for 20 minutes or until rolls are golden. Place baking dish on a wire rack and allow to cool. Divide into 8 servings. Good warm or cold.

Each serving equals:

HE: 1 Bread • ½ Fruit • 16 Optional Calories

133 Calories • 5 gm Fat • 2 gm Protein •
20 gm Carbohydrate • 297 mg Sodium •
10 mg Calcium • 1 gm Fiber

DIABETIC EXCHANGES: 1 Starch • ½ Fruit • ½ Fat

Hawaiian Butterscotch Pie

Do you love butterscotch as much as my daughter does? (I doubt it!) Here's a delightful culinary visit to the islands in one scrumptious pie. ○ Serves 8

> 1 (4-serving) package JELL-O sugar-free instant butterscotch pudding mix
> ⅔ cup Carnation Nonfat Dry Milk Powder
> ½ cup water
> 1 (8-ounce) can crushed pineapple, packed in fruit juice, undrained
> 1 (6-ounce) Keebler graham cracker piecrust
> 1 cup Cool Whip Free
> ½ teaspoon coconut extract
> 2 tablespoons chopped pecans
> 2 tablespoons flaked coconut

In a large bowl, combine dry pudding mix, dry milk powder, water, and undrained pineapple. Mix well using a wire whisk. Spread mixture into piecrust. Refrigerate while preparing topping. In a small bowl, gently combine Cool Whip Free and coconut extract. Evenly spread topping mixture over set filling. Sprinkle pecans and coconut evenly over top. Refrigerate for at least 1 hour. Cut into 8 servings.

Each serving equals:

HE: 1 Bread • ¾ Fat • ¼ Fat-Free Milk • ¼ Fruit • ¼ Slider • 11 Optional Calories

179 Calories • 7 gm Fat • 3 gm Protein • 26 gm Carbohydrate • 344 mg Sodium • 80 mg Calcium • 1 gm Fiber

DIABETIC EXCHANGES: 1½ Starch/Carbohydrate • 1 Fat

Lemon Grove Coconut Cream Pie

I love my garden, where I raise many vegetables and fruits, but sometimes I wonder what it would be like to have an entire orchard of fragrant fruit trees. Here's my hymn to lemons in abundance. As Mae West said, too much of a good thing can be wonderful!

● Serves 8

> 2 (4-serving) packages JELL-O sugar-free instant vanilla pudding
>   mix
> 1 (4-serving) package JELL-O sugar-free lemon gelatin
> 1⅓ cups Carnation Nonfat Dry Milk Powder
> 2½ cups Diet Mountain Dew
> ⅔ cup Cool Whip Free
> 1 teaspoon coconut extract
> ¼ cup flaked coconut ☆
> 1 (6-ounce) Keebler shortbread piecrust

In a large bowl, combine dry pudding mix, dry gelatin, and dry milk powder. Add Diet Mountain Dew. Mix well using a wire whisk. Blend in Cool Whip Free and coconut extract. Stir in 3 tablespoons coconut. Spread mixture into piecrust. Evenly sprinkle remaining coconut over top. Refrigerate for at least 1 hour. Cut into 8 servings.

Each serving equals:

HE: 1 Bread • ½ Fat-Free Milk • ½ Fat • ¼ Slider • 5 Optional Calories

189 Calories • 5 gm Fat • 5 gm Protein • 31 gm Carbohydrate • 531 mg Sodium • 139 mg Calcium • 1 gm Fiber

DIABETIC EXCHANGES: 1½ Starch/Carbohydrate • 1 Fat • ½ Fat-Free Milk

Fort Lauderdale Banana Pie

Iowans dream about Florida during our long, snowy winters, so this recipe is one way I can pretend I'm there, even when the snow is piled high outside the window. I'd serve this en route to the famous Fort Lauderdale Christmas boat parade! ☻ Serves 8

2 cups (2 medium) sliced bananas
1 (6-ounce) Keebler graham cracker piecrust
1 (4-serving) package JELL-O sugar-free instant vanilla pudding
    mix
⅔ cup Carnation Nonfat Dry Milk Powder
1 cup unsweetened orange juice
½ cup Cool Whip Free
1 teaspoon coconut extract
2 tablespoons chopped pecans
2 tablespoons flaked coconut

Layer banana slices in piecrust. In a large bowl, combine dry pudding mix, dry milk powder, and orange juice. Mix well using a wire whisk. Blend in Cool Whip Free and coconut extract. Spread mixture evenly over banana slices. Evenly sprinkle pecans and coconut over top. Refrigerate for at least 1 hour. Cut into 8 servings.

HINT: To prevent bananas from turning brown, mix with 1 teaspoon lemon juice or sprinkle with Fruit Fresh.

Each serving equals:

HE: 1 Bread • ¾ Fruit • ½ Fat • ¼ Fat-Free Milk •
¼ Slider • 4 Optional Calories

---

215 Calories • 7 gm Fat • 4 gm Protein •
34 gm Carbohydrate • 337 mg Sodium •
81 mg Calcium • 2 gm Fiber

DIABETIC EXCHANGES: 1 Starch/Carbohydrate •
1 Fruit • 1 Fat

Razzle Dazzle Banana Cream Pie

What do I mean by calling this yummy-in-the-tummy pie a bit of razzle dazzle? I mean that it's a dessert full of sparkle and sizzle, flavor and fun. One bite, and you'll agree. ◐ Serves 8

2 cups (2 medium) diced bananas
1 (6-ounce) Keebler chocolate piecrust
2 (4-serving) packages JELL-O sugar-free instant banana cream
    pudding mix ☆
1⅓ cups Carnation Nonfat Dry Milk Powder ☆
1¾ cups water ☆
1 (8-ounce) can crushed pineapple, packed in fruit juice, undrained
½ cup Cool Whip Free
2 tablespoons mini chocolate chips

Layer bananas in bottom of piecrust. In a large bowl, combine 1 package dry pudding mix, ⅔ cup dry milk powder, and 1¼ cups water. Mix well using a wire whisk. Pour mixture evenly over bananas. Refrigerate while preparing topping. In a small bowl, combine remaining package dry pudding mix, remaining ⅔ cup dry milk powder, remaining ½ cup water, and undrained pineapple. Mix well using a wire whisk. Blend in Cool Whip Free. Spread topping mixture evenly over pudding layer. Evenly sprinkle chocolate chips over top. Refrigerate for at least 30 minutes. Cut into 8 servings.

HINT: To prevent bananas from turning brown, mix with 1 teaspoon lemon juice or sprinkle with Fruit Fresh.

Each serving equals:

HE: 1 Bread • ¾ Fruit • ½ Fat-Free Milk • ½ Fat •
½ Slider • 2 Optional Calories

242 Calories • 6 gm Fat • 5 gm Protein •
42 gm Carbohydrate • 505 mg Sodium •
146 mg Calcium • 2 gm Fiber

DIABETIC EXCHANGES: 1 Starch/Carbohydrate •
1 Fruit • 1 Fat • ½ Fat-Free Milk

Apple Crumb Pie

There are some kitchen chores the microwave does better than any other appliance, and this recipe makes especially good use of those miraculous rays! You'll find that the fruit doesn't shrink nearly as much as it does in other cooking methods.   ● Serves 8

1 cup unsweetened apple juice
1 teaspoon apple pie spice
3 cups (6 small) cored, unpeeled, and sliced cooking apples
1 (4-serving) package JELL-O sugar-free instant vanilla pudding
    mix
1 (6-ounce) Keebler graham cracker piecrust
6 tablespoons purchased graham cracker crumbs or 6 (2½-inch)
    graham cracker squares, made into crumbs
1 tablespoon Splenda Granular
1 tablespoon + 1 teaspoon reduced-calorie margarine

In an 8-cup glass measuring bowl, combine apple juice and apple pie spice. Stir in sliced apples. Cover and microwave on HIGH (100% power) for 2 to 3 minutes or just until apples are tender. Cool completely for about 20 minutes. Remove apple slices with a slotted spoon. Add dry pudding mix to liquid. Mix well to combine. Stir apple slices back into mixture. Spoon mixture into piecrust. In a small bowl, combine graham cracker crumbs, Splenda, and margarine. Mix well to combine, using a fork. Sprinkle mixture evenly over top of apple mixture. Microwave on HIGH for 60 seconds. Place pie on a wire rack and let set for 1 hour before serving. Cut into 8 servings. Refrigerate leftovers.

Each serving equals:

HE: 1 Bread • 1 Fruit • ½ Fat • ¼ Slider •
11 Optional Calories

---

182 Calories • 6 gm Fat • 1 gm Protein •
31 gm Carbohydrate • 344 mg Sodium •
6 mg Calcium • 2 gm Fiber

DIABETIC EXCHANGES: 1½ Starch/Carbohydrate •
1 Fruit • 1 Fat

No-Bake Lemon Cheesecake Pie

If the temperature's up, here's a wonderful treat that won't heat up your mobile home—it'll just warm your heart and tickle your taste buds. Every bite is oh-so-rich! ❂ Serves 8

1 (4-serving) package JELL-O sugar-free vanilla cook-and-serve
  pudding mix
1 (4-serving) package JELL-O sugar-free lemon gelatin
1⅓ cups water
2 (8-ounce) packages Philadelphia fat-free cream cheese
1 (6-ounce) Keebler graham cracker piecrust
½ cup Cool Whip Lite

In a medium saucepan, combine pudding mix, dry gelatin, and water. Cook over medium heat until mixture thickens and starts to boil, stirring constantly. Remove from heat. Stir in cream cheese. Mix well using a wire whisk, until mixture is well blended. Place saucepan on a wire rack and allow to cool for 10 minutes. Evenly spoon cooled mixture into piecrust. Refrigerate for at least 2 hours. Cut into 8 servings. When serving, top each piece with 1 tablespoon Cool Whip Lite.

HINT: Also good topped with 1 tablespoon spreadable fruit (any fla-
    vor). If using, count calories accordingly.

Each serving equals:

HE: 1 Bread • 1 Protein • ½ Fat • ¼ Slider •
5 Optional Calories

178 Calories • 6 gm Fat • 10 gm Protein •
21 gm Carbohydrate • 469 mg Sodium •
171 mg Calcium • 1 gm Fiber

DIABETIC EXCHANGES: 1 Starch • 1 Meat • 1 Fat

Chocolate Peppermint Cheesecake

If you adore those chocolate-covered peppermint patties (and who doesn't?), here's a delectable sweet that is bound to please! It's marvelously minty, and pretty as well. ❂ Serves 8

> 2 (8-ounce) packages Philadelphia fat-free cream cheese
> 1 (4-serving) package JELL-O sugar-free instant chocolate fudge
>   pudding mix
> ⅔ cup Carnation Nonfat Dry Milk Powder
> 1 cup water
> 1 cup Cool Whip Free ☆
> ½ teaspoon peppermint extract ☆
> 1 (6-ounce) Keebler chocolate piecrust
> 3 to 4 drops red food coloring
> 2 small peppermint hard candies, crushed

In a large bowl, stir cream cheese with a sturdy spoon until soft. Add dry pudding mix, dry milk powder, and water. Mix well using a wire whisk. Blend in ¼ cup Cool Whip Free and ¼ teaspoon peppermint extract. Spread mixture evenly into piecrust. Refrigerate while preparing topping. In a small bowl, combine remaining ¾ cup Cool Whip Free, remaining ¼ teaspoon peppermint extract, and red food coloring. Spread mixture evenly over set filling. Sprinkle crushed candy pieces evenly over top. Refrigerate for at least 1 hour. Cut into 8 servings.

Each serving equals:

HE: 1 Bread • 1 Protein • ½ Fat • ¼ Fat-Free Milk •
¼ Slider • 16 Optional Calories

---

205 Calories • 5 gm Fat • 12 gm Protein •
28 gm Carbohydrate • 526 mg Sodium •
247 mg Calcium • 1 gm Fiber

DIABETIC EXCHANGES: 1½ Starch/Carbohydrate •
1 Meat • 1 Fat

Layered Double Chocolate Cheesecake

Double your pleasure, double your fun—or just double your chocolate intake with this sinfully good dessert! (Actually, it's got two layers of chocolate in a chocolate crust, so it's a true triple threat!)

◐ Serves 8

2 (8-ounce) packages Philadelphia fat-free cream cheese ☆

1 (4-serving) package JELL-O sugar-free instant chocolate fudge pudding mix

1⅓ cups Carnation Nonfat Dry Milk Powder ☆

2 cups water ☆

½ cup Cool Whip Free ☆

1 (6-ounce) Keebler chocolate piecrust

1 (4-serving) package JELL-O sugar-free instant white chocolate pudding mix

1 tablespoon + 1 teaspoon Hershey's Lite Chocolate Syrup

In a large bowl, stir 1 package cream cheese with a sturdy spoon until soft. Add dry chocolate fudge pudding mix, ⅔ cup dry milk powder, and 1 cup water. Mix well using a wire whisk. Blend in ¼ cup Cool Whip Free. Spread mixture into piecrust. Refrigerate while preparing next layer. In another large bowl, stir remaining package of cream cheese with a sturdy spoon until soft. Add dry white chocolate pudding mix, remaining ⅔ cup dry milk powder, and remaining 1 cup water. Blend in remaining ¼ cup Cool Whip Free. Evenly spread mixture over set chocolate layer. Refrigerate for at least 1 hour. Cut into 8 servings. When serving, drizzle ½ teaspoon chocolate syrup over top of each piece.

Each serving equals:

HE: 1 Bread • 1 Protein • ½ Fat-Free Milk • ½ Fat • ½ Slider • 8 Optional Calories

---

233 Calories • 5 gm Fat • 15 gm Protein • 32 gm Carbohydrate • 774 mg Sodium • 323 mg Calcium • 1 gm Fiber

---

DIABETIC EXCHANGES: 1½ Starch/Carbohydrate • 1 Meat • 1 Fat • ½ Fat-Free Milk

Rocky Road White Chocolate Cheesecake

As long as the only rocky road you travel is made of chocolate chips, nuts, and mini-marshmallows, you'll have a very pleasant journey! This is fun food for the whole family, a perfect choice for a birthday party or special event. ❂ Serves 8

2 (8-ounce) packages
  Philadelphia fat-free
  cream cheese
1 (4-serving) package JELL-O
  sugar-free instant white
  chocolate pudding mix
⅔ cup Carnation Nonfat Dry
  Milk Powder
1 cup water

½ cup Cool Whip Free
6 (2½-inch) chocolate graham
  cracker squares, made into
  coarse crumbs
¼ cup chopped walnuts ☆
¼ cup miniature marshmallows
1 (6-ounce) Keebler chocolate
  piecrust
1 tablespoon mini chocolate chips

In a large bowl, stir cream cheese with a sturdy spoon until soft. Add dry pudding mix, dry milk powder, and water. Mix well using a wire whisk. Blend in Cool Whip Free. Add graham cracker crumbs, 3 tablespoons walnuts, and marshmallows. Mix gently to combine. Spread mixture evenly into piecrust. Sprinkle chocolate chips and remaining 1 tablespoon walnuts over top. Refrigerate for at least 1 hour. Cut into 8 servings.

HINT: A self-seal sandwich bag works great for crushing graham crackers.

Each serving equals:

HE: 1 Bread • 1 Protein • ½ Fat • ¼ Fat-Free Milk • ½ Slider • 13 Optional Calories

244 Calories • 8 gm Fat • 12 gm Protein • 31 gm Carbohydrate • 589 mg Sodium • 241 mg Calcium • 1 gm Fiber

DIABETIC EXCHANGES: 1½ Starch/Carbohydrate • 1 Meat • 1 Fat

Romanoff Cheesecake Tarts

These mini-cheesecakes are a great way to show new friends that you're so glad to know them! The fresh strawberries make these extra-special. ☻ Serves 6

> 1 (8-ounce) package Philadelphia fat-free cream cheese
> 1 (4-serving) package JELL-O sugar-free instant vanilla pudding mix
> ⅔ cup Carnation Nonfat Dry Milk Powder
> ½ cup unsweetened orange juice
> ½ cup water
> ¾ cup Cool Whip Free
> 1 cup finely chopped fresh strawberries
> 1 (6 single-serve) package Keebler graham cracker crusts

In a large bowl, stir cream cheese with a sturdy spoon until soft. Add dry pudding mix, dry milk powder, orange juice, and water. Mix well using a wire whisk. Blend in Cool Whip Free. Add strawberries. Mix gently to combine. Evenly spoon filling mixture into crusts. Refrigerate for at least 1 hour.

Each serving equals:

HE: 1 Bread • ⅔ Protein • ½ Fat • ⅓ Fat-Free Milk • ⅓ Fruit • ¼ Slider • 12 Optional Calories

222 Calories • 6 gm Fat • 10 gm Protein • 32 gm Carbohydrate • 599 mg Sodium • 213 mg Calcium • 1 gm Fiber

DIABETIC EXCHANGES: 1½ Starch/Carbohydrate • 1 Meat • 1 Fat

Express Extras

It's the little things that make life not only bearable but full of pleasure and fun, don't you agree? With the goodies in this chapter, you can throw together a tasty tailgate party when your route includes an unplanned stop at a high school football game! You can turn your RV kitchen into a mobile takeout shop, cooking up calzones and quesadillas whenever you like. (Cliff doesn't like to hit the road until he's sure I've packed bags of party mix and popcorn treats for those munchie attacks that seem to happen every couple of hundred miles!)

You'll discover how easy it is to entertain the Healthy Exchanges way with the dips, drinks, and other delights in this section. Why eat plain old raw veggies when you can make them sparkle by dunking them in **Ranch Cheddar and Bacon Dip**? And instead of plain hard-boiled eggs for your next picnic, try my **Dilled Ham Deviled Eggs**— and enjoy the compliments you get! I'm especially proud of my fun and fizzy drink recipes that are party-perfect, and just right for everyone age nine to ninety. (The **Ruby Slipper** is so pretty in pink!) Whether you've got a hankering for pizza treats or cheesy scones, you'll find just what you're looking for here.

Express Extras

Peanut Butter Popcorn Treats

For those times when good enough just isn't great enough, here's a super-duper snack that no one will be able to resist. It's a good idea to make this for a crowd, so you won't be quite as tempted to gobble up the entire batch. **☉** Serves 9 (1 cup)

9 cups air-popped popcorn
¼ cup + 2 tablespoons reduced-fat peanut butter
2 tablespoons I Can't Believe It's Not Butter! Light Margarine

Preheat oven to 375 degrees. Place popped popcorn in a very large bowl. In a small saucepan, melt peanut butter and margarine over low heat, stirring constantly until smooth. Drizzle melted mixture over popcorn. Mix well to coat. Spray large baking sheet or jelly roll pan with butter-flavored cooking spray. Evenly spread popcorn mixture in pan. Bake for 4 to 6 minutes, stirring every 2 minutes.

HINT: Usually a full ½ cup unpopped corn makes about 9 cups popped popcorn, if prepared in an air popper.

Each serving equals:

HE: 1 Fat • ⅔ Protein • ⅓ Bread

101 Calories • 5 gm Fat • 4 gm Protein •
10 gm Carbohydrate • 89 mg Sodium •
6 mg Calcium • 2 gm Fiber

DIABETIC EXCHANGES: 1 Fat • ½ Meat • ½ Starch

Cajun Party Mix

It's a great idea to have bags of healthy snacks ready for those times when the munchies strike. Otherwise, you're likely to grab the nearest high-fat chips and cookies you can find. This is one of Cliff's favorite blends, and once you taste it, you'll know just why.

☻ Serves 8 (1 full cup)

> 6 cups air-popped popcorn
> 2 teaspoons Cajun seasoning
> 1½ cups Corn Chex
> 2 cups coarsely crushed lightly salted pretzels

Lightly spray hot popcorn with butter-flavored cooking spray. In a large bowl, combine popcorn and Cajun seasoning. Add Corn Chex and pretzels. Mix well to combine.

HINT: Usually 4 tablespoons unpopped corn makes about 6 cups popped popcorn, if prepared in an air popper.

Each serving equals:

HE: 1 Bread

---

64 Calories • 0 gm Fat • 2 gm Protein •
14 gm Carbohydrate • 498 mg Sodium •
20 mg Calcium • 1 gm Fiber

DIABETIC EXCHANGES: 1 Starch

Pineapple Dip

Instead of just snacking on slices of fresh fruit, why not serve it with a creamy fruit dip that makes it feel extra special? Even if it's just a party for one, you deserve a treat! 〇 Serves 8 (¼ cup)

1 (8-ounce) package Philadelphia fat-free cream cheese
1 (8-ounce) can crushed pineapple, packed in fruit juice, drained
1 tablespoon Splenda Granular
¼ cup (1 ounce) chopped pecans
1 cup Cool Whip Free

In a medium bowl, stir cream cheese with a sturdy spoon until soft. Add pineapple, Splenda, and pecans. Mix well to combine. Stir in Cool Whip Free. Cover and refrigerate for at least 30 minutes. Gently stir again just before serving.

HINT: Good with fresh fruit.

Each serving equals:

HE: ½ Protein • ½ Fat • ¼ Fruit •
16 Optional Calories

66 Calories • 2 gm Fat • 5 gm Protein •
7 gm Carbohydrate • 143 mg Sodium •
92 mg Calcium • 1 gm Fiber

DIABETIC EXCHANGES: ½ Meat • ½ Fat •
½ Starch/Carbohydrate

Banana Plantation Dip

This creamy blend is a true taste of the tropics, ideal for dunking chunks of fresh fruit or even a Healthy Exchanges cookie if you're feeling really wild. Where is that old fondue set? You could use those long forks to dip without losing your grip!

☻ Serves 8 (⅓ cup)

> 1 (4-serving) package JELL-O sugar-free instant banana cream
>   pudding mix
> ⅔ cup Carnation Nonfat Dry Milk Powder
> 1⅔ cups water
> 1 cup Cool Whip Free
> 1 teaspoon rum extract

In a large bowl, combine dry pudding mix, dry milk powder, and water. Mix well using a wire whisk. Blend in Cool Whip Free and rum extract. Cover and refrigerate for at least 30 minutes. Gently stir again just before serving.

HINT: Wonderful with fresh pineapple, kiwi fruit, or apples.

Each serving equals:

HE: ¼ Fat-Free Milk • ¼ Slider • 8 Optional Calories

---

44 Calories • 0 gm Fat • 2 gm Protein •
9 gm Carbohydrate • 206 mg Sodium •
75 mg Calcium • 0 gm Fiber

DIABETIC EXCHANGES: ½ Starch/Carbohydrate

French Cheese Dip

Let's party til the cows come home, as the saying goes—or at least til the sun goes down and the moon rises! Make those plain old raw veggies a crudite celebration with this cheesy, tangy dip.

❍   Serves 4 (¼ cup)

> 1 (8-ounce) package Philadelphia fat-free cream cheese
> 3 tablespoons Kraft Fat Free French Dressing
> 1 tablespoon Worcestershire sauce
> dash of garlic salt

In a medium bowl, stir cream cheese with a sturdy spoon until soft. Add French dressing, Worcestershire sauce, and garlic salt. Mix well until smooth. Cover and refrigerate for at least 30 minutes. Gently stir again just before serving.

HINT: Good served with raw vegetables.

Each serving equals:

HE: 1 Protein • 10 Optional Calories

72 Calories • 0 gm Fat • 9 gm Protein •
9 gm Carbohydrate • 437 mg Sodium •
176 mg Calcium • 0 gm Fiber

DIABETIC EXCHANGES: 1 Meat

Ranch Cheddar and Bacon Dip

Are you the kind of person who watches TV, works at your computer, and nibbles at your lunch? Well, then, this is your kind of dip, with three strong flavors that combine for an extravaganza of delight.

☻ Serves 6 (¼ cup)

> ¾ cup Land O Lakes no-fat sour cream
> ¼ cup Kraft Fat Free Ranch Dressing
> 2 teaspoons dried onion flakes
> 1 tablespoon dried parsley flakes
> ½ cup + 1 tablespoon (2¼ ounces) shredded Kraft reduced-fat
>   Cheddar cheese
> 3 tablespoons Hormel Bacon Bits

In a medium bowl, combine sour cream, Ranch dressing, onion flakes, and parsley flakes. Add Cheddar cheese and bacon bits. Mix gently to combine. Cover and refrigerate for at least 30 minutes. Gently stir again just before serving.

HINT: Good on crackers, with vegetables, or spread on a hot baked potato.

Each serving equals:

HE: ½ Protein • ½ Slider • 19 Optional Calories

---

82 Calories • 2 gm Fat • 6 gm Protein •
10 gm Carbohydrate • 374 mg Sodium •
112 mg Calcium • 0 gm Fiber

DIABETIC EXCHANGES: ½ Meat •
½ Starch/Carbohydrate

Apple Walnut Spread

Why pay extra to purchase those special spreads from the bagel shop, when you can stir up such fresh and tasty versions of your own? Make your weekend brunch a true meal to remember with this topper.   ☻   Serves 6 (¼ cup)

> 1 (8-ounce) package Philadelphia fat-free cream cheese
> 2 tablespoons Log Cabin Sugar Free Maple Syrup
> 2 tablespoons Splenda Granular
> 1 cup (2 small) cored, peeled, and finely chopped Red Delicious apples
> ¼ cup (1 ounce) chopped walnuts

In a medium bowl, stir cream cheese with a sturdy spoon until soft. Stir in maple syrup and Splenda. Add apples and walnuts. Mix well to combine. Cover and refrigerate for at least 30 minutes. Gently stir again just before serving.

HINT: Great with crackers or as a sandwich filling.

Each serving equals:

> HE: ⅔ Protein • ⅓ Fruit • ⅓ Fat •
> 12 Optional Calories
> _____
> 83 Calories • 3 gm Fat • 6 gm Protein •
> 8 gm Carbohydrate • 195 mg Sodium •
> 120 mg Calcium • 1 gm Fiber
> _____
> DIABETIC EXCHANGES: 1 Meat • ½ Fat •
> ½ Starch/Carbohydrate

Tuna and Olive Spread

Planning a party or potluck but can't decide what to serve? Here's a savory spread that is sure to please your guests and provide a delightful accompaniment to raw veggies and crackers.

☻ Serves 6 (⅓ cup)

> 1 (8-ounce) package Philadelphia fat-free cream cheese
> 2 tablespoons Land O Lakes no-fat sour cream
> 2 teaspoons dried onion flakes
> 1 teaspoon dried parsley flakes
> ⅛ teaspoon black pepper
> 1 (6-ounce) can white tuna, packed in water, drained and flaked
> 1 hard-boiled egg, finely chopped
> ⅓ cup chopped ripe olives

In a large bowl, stir cream cheese with a sturdy spoon until soft. Add sour cream, onion flakes, parsley flakes, and black pepper. Mix well to combine. Fold in tuna, chopped egg, and olives. Cover and refrigerate for at least 1 hour. Gently stir again just before serving.

HINT: Great with crackers, fresh veggies, or as a sandwich filling.

Each serving equals:

HE: 1½ Protein • ¼ Fat • 10 Optional Calories

---

94 Calories • 2 gm Fat • 14 gm Protein •
5 gm Carbohydrate • 376 mg Sodium •
144 mg Calcium • 0 gm Fiber

DIABETIC EXCHANGES: 1½ Meat • ½ Fat

Mushroom Marinara Sauce

Here's a handy homemade sauce you can spoon over pasta or vegetables. It's just another of the great ways you can choose to use ready-made healthy salad dressing.   ○   Serves 4 (⅔ cup)

½ *cup chopped onion*
¼ *cup Kraft Fat Free Italian Dressing*
3 *cups peeled and chopped fresh tomatoes*
1½ *cups chopped fresh mushrooms*
2 *tablespoons Splenda Granular*

In a large skillet sprayed with olive oil–flavored cooking spray, sauté onion for 5 minutes. Add Italian dressing, tomatoes, and mushrooms. Mix well to combine. Stir in Splenda. Lower heat and simmer for 15 to 20 minutes, stirring occasionally.

Each serving equals:

HE: 2½ Vegetable • 9 Optional Calories

57 Calories • 1 gm Fat • 2 gm Protein •
10 gm Carbohydrate • 239 mg Sodium •
12 mg Calcium • 2 gm Fiber

DIABETIC EXCHANGES: 2 Vegetable

Dilled Ham Deviled Eggs

For those all-summer-long, side-of-the-road picnics, try these festive deviled delights. So little dill makes such a great big taste difference—you'll see what I mean! ☺ Serves 4 (2 halves)

4 hard-boiled eggs
3 tablespoons Kraft fat-free mayonnaise
1 teaspoon prepared yellow mustard
¼ teaspoon dried dill weed
¼ cup (1½ ounces) finely diced Dubuque 97% fat-free ham or any
*   extra-lean ham*

Cut eggs in half lengthwise and remove yolks. Place yolks in a medium bowl and mash well using a fork. Add mayonnaise, mustard, dill weed, and ham. Mix well to combine. Refill egg white halves by spooning 1 full tablespoon filling mixture into each half. Cover and refrigerate for at least 30 minutes.

Each serving equals:

HE: 1¼ Protein • 7 Optional Calories

85 Calories • 5 gm Fat • 8 gm Protein •
2 gm Carbohydrate • 210 mg Sodium •
26 mg Calcium • 0 gm Fiber

DIABETIC EXCHANGES: 1 Meat

Toasted Shrimp Treats

If you want to show your guests how much their presence means to you, these pretty hors d'oeuvres are just about perfect! Make sure you get to taste at least one or two while you're playing hostess.

● Serves 6 (4 each)

> ½ cup Kraft fat-free mayonnaise
> 1 teaspoon prepared yellow mustard
> 1 teaspoon dried onion flakes
> 1 teaspoon dried parsley flakes
> 1 (4.5-ounce drained weight) can small shrimp, rinsed and drained
> ¼ cup + 2 teaspoons (1⅛ ounces) shredded Kraft reduced-fat
>   Cheddar cheese
> 24 pumpernickel bread rounds or squares

Preheat oven to 425 degrees. Spray 2 baking sheets with butter-flavored cooking spray. In a medium bowl, combine mayonnaise, mustard, onion flakes, and parsley flakes. Stir in shrimp and Cheddar cheese. Spread 2 teaspoons shrimp mixture over each bread round. Place rounds on prepared baking sheets. Bake for 5 minutes. Serve hot.

Each serving equals:

HE: 1 Bread • 1 Protein • 13 Optional Calories

151 Calories • 3 gm Fat • 10 gm Protein •
21 gm Carbohydrate • 497 mg Sodium •
78 mg Calcium • 2 gm Fiber

DIABETIC EXCHANGES: 1 Starch • 1 Meat

Bacon-Cheese Pizza Treats

Usually, it's the kids who get to enjoy English muffin pizzas, but why should the young have all the fun? These savory specialties have your name on them!   ☻   Serves 6

> *3 English muffins, halved and toasted*
> *1 (8-ounce) can Hunt's Tomato Sauce*
> *6 tablespoons Hormel Bacon Bits*
> *1 teaspoon dried parsley flakes*
> *2 teaspoons Splenda Granular*
> *¾ cup (3 ounces) shredded Kraft reduced-fat Cheddar cheese*

Preheat oven to 415 degrees. Spray a baking sheet with butter-flavored cooking spray. Arrange muffin halves on prepared baking sheet. In a small bowl, combine tomato sauce, bacon bits, parsley flakes, and Splenda. Spread 3 full tablespoons sauce mixture over each muffin half. Sprinkle 2 tablespoons Cheddar cheese over top of each. Bake for 10 minutes. Serve hot.

Each serving equals:

HE: 1 Bread • ⅔ Protein • ⅔ Vegetable • ¼ Slider •
6 Optional Calories

---

140 Calories • 4 gm Fat • 9 gm Protein •
17 gm Carbohydrate • 748 mg Sodium •
150 mg Calcium • 1 gm Fiber

DIABETIC EXCHANGES: 1 Starch • 1 Meat • ½ Vegetable

Creamy Quesadilla Snacks

If your family loves Mexican-style goodies but you've never made them at home, maybe it's time to give these easy snacks a try! Make sure you use reduced-fat cheese, not fat-free, so it melts beautifully every time.   ❂   Serves 4

½ cup (4 ounces) Philadelphia fat-free cream cheese
½ cup chunky salsa (mild, medium, or hot)
⅓ cup (1½ ounces) shredded Kraft reduced-fat Cheddar cheese
4 (6-inch) flour tortillas

In a medium bowl, stir cream cheese with a sturdy spoon until soft. Stir in salsa and Cheddar cheese. Spread about ¼ cup mixture on each tortilla. Fold tortillas in half. Place tortillas in a large skillet sprayed with olive oil–flavored cooking spray and lightly brown tortillas for 2 to 3 minutes on each side. Serve warm.

Each serving equals:

HE: 1 Bread • 1 Protein • ¼ Vegetable

181 Calories • 5 gm Fat • 11 gm Protein •
23 gm Carbohydrate • 504 mg Sodium •
211 mg Calcium • 2 gm Fiber

DIABETIC EXCHANGES: 1 Starch • 1 Meat

Personal Calzone Treats

Even if you're out in the middle of nowhere, without a pizza place anywhere near, you can still satisfy your craving for delicious calzones—and you know you're living healthy at the same time!

● Serves 5 (1 each)

> 1 (7.5-ounce) can Pillsbury refrigerated buttermilk biscuits
> 1/2 cup reduced-sodium ketchup
> 2 tablespoons water
> 1 teaspoon Italian seasoning
> 1 tablespoon Splenda Granular
> 1 (2.5-ounce) jar sliced mushrooms, drained
> 1/2 cup + 1 tablespoon (2¼ ounces) shredded Kraft reduced-fat
>   Cheddar cheese
> 1/3 cup (1½ ounces) shredded Kraft reduced-fat mozzarella cheese

Preheat oven to 425 degrees. Spray a baking sheet with olive oil–flavored cooking spray. Separate and flatten biscuits. Place 5 flattened biscuits on prepared baking sheet. In a medium bowl, combine ketchup, water, Italian seasoning, Splenda, mushrooms, Cheddar cheese, and mozzarella cheese. Evenly spoon sauce mixture over biscuits. Carefully arrange a flattened biscuit over top of each. Using the tines of a fork, seal edges. Lightly spray tops with olive oil–flavored cooking spray. Bake for 6 to 8 minutes or until biscuits are golden brown. Place baking sheet on a wire rack and let set for 2 to 3 minutes. Serve hot.

Each serving equals:

HE: 1½ Bread • 1 Protein • ¼ Slider •
4 Optional Calories

---

189 Calories • 5 gm Fat • 9 gm Protein •
27 gm Carbohydrate • 568 mg Sodium •
145 mg Calcium • 3 gm Fiber

DIABETIC EXCHANGES: 1½ Starch • 1 Meat

Cheese Scone Snacks

You may find yourself baking more "on the road" than you do at home, now that you've got such quick and easy recipes to try. These make a great addition for Sunday brunch or with a salad for lunch.
● Serves 8

> 1½ cups Bisquick Reduced Fat Baking Mix
> 2 tablespoons Splenda Granular
> ⅓ cup (1½ ounces) shredded Kraft reduced-fat Cheddar cheese
> 1 teaspoon dried parsley flakes
> ½ cup Land O Lakes no-fat sour cream
> ½ teaspoon prepared yellow mustard

Preheat oven to 400 degrees. Spray a 9-by-9-inch cake pan with butter-flavored cooking spray. In a large bowl, combine baking mix, Splenda, Cheddar cheese, and parsley flakes. Add sour cream and mustard. Mix well to combine. Divide mixture evenly into 8 portions. Spray hands with butter-flavored cooking spray and shape each section into a ball. Place balls in prepared cake pan. Bake for 15 to 20 minutes or until lightly browned. Place cake pan on a wire rack and let set for 5 minutes.

Each serving equals:

HE: 1 Bread • ¼ Protein • 17 Optional Calories

---

106 Calories • 2 gm Fat • 3 gm Protein •
19 gm Carbohydrate • 329 mg Sodium •
78 mg Calcium • 1 gm Fiber

DIABETIC EXCHANGES: 1 Starch

Tropical Smoothie

Want a great way to get those needed servings of good-for-you fruits? A smoothie is soul-satisfying and tummy-filling, especially when you choose a fruity soda for the liquid component.

○ Serves 4 (1 cup)

> *1 cup (1 medium) diced banana*
> *1 (8-ounce) can crushed pineapple, packed in fruit juice, undrained*
> *2 cups cold Diet Mountain Dew*
> *1 (4-serving) package JELL-O sugar-free strawberry gelatin*

In a blender container, combine diced banana, undrained pineapple, and Diet Mountain Dew. Cover and process on BLEND for 10 seconds. Add dry gelatin. Re-cover and continue processing on BLEND for 15 to 20 seconds or until mixture is smooth. Pour into tall glasses filled with ice and serve at once.

Each serving equals:

HE: 1 Fruit • 10 Optional Calories

---

56 Calories • 0 gm Fat • 1 gm Protein •
13 gm Carbohydrate • 11 mg Sodium •
11 mg Calcium • 1 gm Fiber

DIABETIC EXCHANGES: 1 Fruit

Ruby Slipper

The shoes were lucky for Dorothy on her journey to Oz, so I hope this lovely beverage will bring you happy times and the cozy comfort of feeling you're home, no matter where you hang your hat.

◐ Serves 4 (1 cup)

3 cups Ocean Spray reduced-calorie cranberry juice cocktail
1 cup Diet Rite white grape soda pop or Diet 7-UP
½ teaspoon lime juice

In a pitcher, combine cranberry juice cocktail, grape soda pop, and lime juice. Mix well to combine. Pour into tall glasses filled with ice and serve at once.

Each serving equals:

HE: ¾ Fruit

---

40 Calories • 0 gm Fat • 0 gm Protein •
10 gm Carbohydrate • 40 mg Sodium • 0 mg Calcium •
0 gm Fiber

DIABETIC EXCHANGES: 1 Fruit

Orange Dew Spritzer

It takes two to tango, as the saying goes. Well, here's a drink that tastes as delectable as dancing the night away feels!

☻ Serves 4 (1 cup)

2 cups cold unsweetened orange juice
2 cups cold Diet Mountain Dew

In a pitcher, combine orange juice and Diet Mountain Dew. Pour into 4 tall glasses filled with ice and serve at once.

Each serving equals:

HE: 1 Fruit

48 Calories • 0 gm Fat • 0 gm Protein • 12 gm Carbohydrate • 15 mg Sodium • 10 mg Calcium • 0 gm Fiber

DIABETIC EXCHANGES: 1 Fruit

Designated Driver's Champagne

This fun and fizzy combo will create a festive mood, even if there's not a drop of alcohol on the premises! Drop a strawberry into the bottom of each champagne flute (glass) and you'll feel like Cinderella at the ball. ☺   Serves 4 (1 cup)

2 cups cold unsweetened apple cider
2 cups cold diet ginger ale

In a pitcher, combine apple cider and diet ginger ale. Pour into 4 champagne glasses. Serve at once.

Each serving equals:

HE: 1 Fruit

---

56 Calories • 0 gm Fat • 0 gm Protein •
14 gm Carbohydrate • 25 mg Sodium •
9 mg Calcium • 0 gm Fiber

DIABETIC EXCHANGES: 1 Fruit

Campsite Coffee Mix

Pre-mixing this deliciously spiced coffee/chocolate blend is such a great idea, even if I did think of it myself! All you need for a special hot drink is a cup of boiling water and a spoonful of this—enjoy!

1 cup Nesquik sugar-free chocolate drink mix
½ cup instant coffee crystals
1 cup Coffee-mate fat-free non-dairy creamer
¾ cup Splenda Granular
1 teaspoon ground cinnamon
½ teaspoon ground nutmeg

In a large bowl, combine chocolate drink mix, coffee crystals, and creamer. Stir in Splenda, cinnamon, and nutmeg. Pour mixture into a blender container. Cover and process on BLEND for 15 to 20 seconds. Store in an airtight container. When using, stir 1 tablespoon mixture into 1 cup boiling water.

1 tablespoon equals:

HE: 12 Optional Calories

---

12 Calories • 0 gm Fat • 0 gm Protein • 3 gm Carbohydrate • 8 mg Sodium • 1 mg Calcium • 0 gm Fiber

---

DIABETIC EXCHANGES: Free Food

A Melange of
Roadside Menus

You've stocked the fridge and pantry, gassed up the motor home, and mapped out your journey—but when your family says, "What's for dinner?" you often feel stumped. Planning meals when you're on the road is not only a good idea, it streamlines your preparation, cuts the time spent in the kitchen and the grocery store, and frees you up to enjoy the benefits of whatever part of the country you're currently visiting. So here are some ideas for easy, speedy, tasty meals the whole gang will love.

Backroads Brunch

Denver Brunch Bake

Apple Pancakes

Yummy Cinnamon Breakfast Squares

Campsite Coffee Mix

"It's Time for a Tailgate" Party

Hot Dog Wraps

BBQ Turkey Sandwiches

A Big Bunch of Potato Salad

Pecan Delight Dessert Pizza

"Pining for a Home-Cooked Meal" Supper

South of the Border Macaroni and Cheese

Tomato Basil Meat Loaf

Green Bean and Bacon Bake

Cinnamon Cherry Cobbler

"Let's Pull Over by the Side of the Road" Picnic

Creamy Coleslaw

Hawaiian Ham Pasta Salad

Eggcellent Egg Salad Sandwiches

Triple Treat Chocolate Cake Brownies

A "Delectable Detour" Sunday Lunch for New Friends

Toasted Shrimp Treats

Layered Tomato Casserole

Celery Stroganoff over English Muffins

Razzle Dazzle Banana Cream Pie

"Safe from the Storm" Cozy Candlelight Dinner

Corn and Chicken Noodle Soup

Honey Mustard Chicken–Potato Bake

Unbelievably Good Green Beans

Chocolate Velvet Ribbon Dessert

Making Healthy Exchanges® Work for You

You're ready now to begin a wonderful journey to better health. In the preceding pages, you've discovered the remarkable variety of good food available to you when you begin eating the Healthy Exchanges way. You've stocked your pantry and learned many of my food preparation "secrets" that will point you on the way to delicious success.

But before I let you go, I'd like to share a few tips that I've learned while traveling toward healthier eating habits. It took me a long time to learn how to eat *smarter*. In fact, I'm still working on it. But I am getting better. For years, I could *inhale* a five-course meal in five minutes flat—and still make room for a second helping of dessert!

Now, I follow certain signposts on the road that help me stay on the right path. I hope these ideas will help point you in the right direction as well.

1. **Eat slowly** so your brain has time to catch up with your tummy. Cut and chew each bite slowly. Try putting your fork down between bites. Stop eating as soon as you feel full. Crumple your napkin and throw it on top of your plate so you don't continue to eat when you are no longer hungry.

2. **Smaller plates** may help you feel more satisfied by your food portions *and* limit the amount you can put on the plate.

3. **Watch portion size.** If you are *truly* hungry, you can always add more food to your plate once you've finished your initial

serving. But remember to count the additional food accordingly.

4. **Always eat at your dining-room or kitchen table.** You deserve better than nibbling from an open refrigerator or over the sink. Make an attractive place setting, even if you're eating alone. Feed your eyes as well as your stomach. By always eating at a table, you will become much more aware of your true food intake. For some reason, many of us conveniently "forget" the food we swallow while standing over the stove or munching in the car or on the run.

5. **Avoid doing anything else while you are eating.** If you read the paper or watch television while you eat, it's easy to consume too much food without realizing it, because you are concentrating on something else besides what you're eating. Then, when you look down at your plate and see that it's empty, you wonder where all the food went and why you still feel hungry.

Day by day, as you travel the path to good health, it will become easier to make the right choices, to eat *smarter*. But don't ever fool yourself into thinking that you'll be able to put your eating habits on cruise control and forget about them. Making a commitment to eat good healthy food and sticking to it takes some effort. But with all the good-tasting recipes in this Healthy Exchanges cookbook, just think how well you're going to eat—and enjoy it—from now on!

Healthy Lean Bon Appetit!

Index

Page numbers in **bold** indicate tables.

We want to hear from you . . .

The love of JoAnna's life was creating "common folk" healthy recipes and solving everyday cooking questions in *The Healthy Exchanges Way*. Everyone who uses her recipes is considered part of the Healthy Exchanges family, so please write to Cliff and Gina if you have any questions, comments, or suggestions. We will do our best to answer. With your support, Healthy Exchanges will continue to provide recipes and cooking tips for many years to come.

Write to: Clifford Lund
c/o Healthy Exchanges, Inc.
P.O. Box 80
DeWitt, IA 52742-0080

If you prefer, you can fax us at 1-563-659-2126 or contact us via e-mail by writing to HealthyJo@aol.com. Or visit our Healthy Exchanges Internet website at www.healthyexchanges.com.

Ever since I began stirring up Healthy Exchanges recipes, I wanted every dish to be rich in flavor and lively in taste. As part of my pursuit of satisfying eating and healthy living for a lifetime, I decided to create my own line of spices.

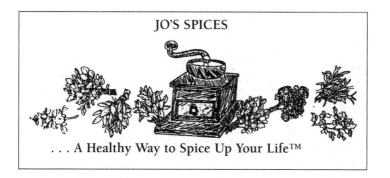

JO'S SPICES

. . . A Healthy Way to Spice Up Your Life™

JO's Spices are salt-, sugar-, wheat-, and MSG-free, and you can substitute them in any of the recipes calling for traditional spice mixes. If you're interested in hearing more about my special blends, please call Healthy Exchanges at 1-563-659-8234 for more information or to order. If you prefer, write to JO's Spices, c/o Healthy Exchanges, P.O. Box 80, DeWitt, IA 52742-0080.

Now That You've Seen *The Open Road Cookbook*, Why Not Order *The Healthy Exchanges Food Newsletter?*

If you enjoyed the recipes in this cookbook and would like to cook up even more of my "common folk" healthy dishes, you may want to subscribe to *The Healthy Exchanges Food Newsletter.*

This monthly 12-page newsletter contains 30-plus new recipes *every month* in such columns as:

- From Our Readers
- Plug It In
- Dinner for Two
- Meatless Main Dishes
- Rise & Shine
- Our Small World
- Brown Bagging It
- Snack Attack
- Side Dishes
- Main Dishes
- Desserts

In addition to all the recipes, other regular features include:

- The Editor's Motivational Corner
- Ask Anything
- Cookbook Classics
- New Product Alert
- Exercise Advice from a Cardiac Rehab Specialist
- Nutrition Advice from a Registered Dietitian
- Positive Thought for the Month

The cost for a one-year (12-issue) subscription is $25. To order, call our toll-free number and pay with any major credit card—or send a check to the address on page iv of this book.

1-800-766-8961 for Customer Orders
1-563-659-8234 for Customer Service

Thank you for your order and for choosing to become a part of the Healthy Exchanges Family!